# Challenging Cases in Pleural Diseases

Although we live in an era of evidence-based medicine, case histories have always had an important role in medical education. This book aims to provide complex case-based learning in pleural medicine, which is an integral part of respiratory medicine. It delivers practical knowledge learned through the experience of leading international authorities. Each case comprises clinical history, investigation, diagnosis, management and detailed answers with discussion and key points. These interesting/challenging/puzzling real case histories will stimulate the reader's mind with interactive questions and answers, imparting in-depth knowledge in the diagnosis and management of complex pleural cases.

## KEY FEATURES

- Contains high-quality illustrations of challenging cases to aid learning for speciality and certification exams
- Serves as an invaluable resource for pulmonologists, radiologists, critical care physicians and trainees
- First case history–based book to be published exclusively for pleural medicine

T0134096

# Challenging Cases in Pleural Diseases

Edited by
Professor Najib M Rahman
Dr Radhika Banka

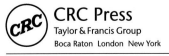

CRC Press
Taylor & Francis Group
Boca Raton London New York

CRC Press is an imprint of the
Taylor & Francis Group, an **informa** business

Cover image: Shutterstock ID 2121207512

First edition published 2024
by CRC Press
6000 Broken Sound Parkway NW, Suite 300, Boca Raton, FL 33487-2742

and by CRC Press
4 Park Square, Milton Park, Abingdon, Oxon, OX14 4RN
*CRC Press is an imprint of Taylor & Francis Group, LLC*

ISBN: 9780367533724 (hbk)
ISBN: 9780367533717 (pbk)
ISBN: 9781003081630 (ebk)

DOI: 10.1201/9781003081630

Typeset in Minion
by Deanta Global Publishing Services, Chennai, India

# Dedication

We would like to acknowledge our patients – whether their cases are listed in this book or not. It is truly a privilege to practice medicine, and we have learnt so much from them; from their diagnoses, response to treatment and management, and perhaps more importantly from their patience and dignity in the face of the most profound challenges and difficulty.

# Contents

Preface                                                                            ix

Editors                                                                             x

Contributors                                                                        xi

1   A post-operative pleural effusion                                               1
    *Anand Sundaralingam*
2   Pleural effusion and chest pain in an elderly gentleman                         10
    *Mohamed Ellayeh*
3   A difficult-to-drain effusion                                                   18
    *Vineeth George*
4   A recurrent and persistent effusion                                            25
    *Eihab Bedawi*
5   To ambulate or admit?                                                          33
    *Eihab Bedawi*
6   Right-sided pleural effusion in a young Nepalese man                           41
    *Radhika Banka*
7   Bilateral transudative effusions                                               46
    *Poppy Denniston*
8   Renal failure and pleural fluid                                                52
    *Anand Sundaralingam*
9   Management of pleural effusion in a patient with known liver disease           58
    *Mohamed Ellayeh*
10  Pleural effusion and thickening after asbestos exposure                        64
    *Hui Guo*
11  Recurrent effusion in a cyclist                                                70
    *Dinesh Addala*
12  Pleural thickening and effusion in a traveller                                 76
    *Hui Guo*
13  Recurrent effusion in a patient on amiodarone                                  84
    *Najib M Rahman*

14  A case of green pleural fluid                                          91
    *Rachelle Asciak*
15  Pleural effusion in a patient with previous pancreatitis               95
    *Vineeth George*
16  Pleural effusion and abnormal bones                                   101
    *Najib M Rahman*
17  Pleural effusion in a patient with chronic myeloid leukaemia          107
    *Dinesh Addala*
18  An unusual pleural abnormality                                        112
    *Rachelle Asciak*
19  Pneumothorax in chronic lung disease                                  116
    *Beenish Iqbal*
20  Air in the wrong place                                                124
    *Rob Hallifax*
21  Recurrent chest pain in a young woman                                 129
    *Beenish Iqbal*
22  An interesting case of recurrent pneumothoraces                       136
    *Rob Hallifax*
23  Post-effusion drainage complication in an 86-year-old woman           142
    *Poppy Denniston*
24  Chest pain in a 65-year-old writer following pleural fluid aspiration 147
    *Soumya Ghatak and Radhika Banka*
25  A simple pneumothorax?                                                153
    *Rachel Mercer*

Index                                                                     159

# Preface

Patients are the best teachers for doctors; each patient provides new depths of learning and insight if the clinician is attuned to these opportunities.

Although we rightly live in an era of evidence-based medicine, individual case experiences form an essential part of our day-to-day learning, as they enhance awareness of rare diseases and unusual presentations and provide a real-world framework in which to apply evidence. With this in mind, it gives us great pleasure to present *Challenging Cases in Pleural Diseases*, which is a compilation of 25 interesting and yet difficult cases in pleural medicine that we have encountered over the past few years at the Oxford Pleural Unit.

Pleural medicine is a subspeciality in its own right, with its own evidence base and clinical expertise – with a wonderful balance of the acute and chronic, interventional and academic, requirement for thought or swift action. Each case has thus been compiled in an interactive form, with a short history and relevant questions and subsequent answers for the readers, to cover these diverse skills. Most of the cases have had a detailed work-up, including radiology and histopathology. Each chapter ends with a list of salient learning points which the authors thought were most relevant. The case-based approach demonstrates potential pitfalls when dealing with such clinical scenarios, focuses on the authors' line of evaluation and treatment, and provides discussion and learning points.

We hope these cases will stimulate the reader and provide insight and knowledge to undergraduates, postgraduates and practising physicians.

We would like to express our thanks to the various authors for their valuable time in order to contribute to this book. This book would not have seen the light of day without the untiring efforts of the team of Taylor & Francis Group, including Shivangi Pramanik and Himani Dwivedi, in going through proofs and pushing us to publish!

# Editors

**Najib M Rahman** is a Consultant Respiratory Physician at the Oxford University Hospitals NHS Foundation Trust, UK, and is Director of the Oxford Respiratory Trials Unit, University of Oxford (Churchill Hospital, Oxford, UK). Having qualified in Oxford, he underwent his medical senior house officer rotation at Queen's Medical Centre (Nottingham, UK) and rejoined Oxford as a specialist registrar in 2003. He undertook a DPhil and MSc during this period and was appointed as consultant and lead for pleural disease in Oxford in 2011. He was appointed as an associate professor in 2014 and a professor of respiratory medicine in 2018.

He has been involved in major randomised controlled trials and observational studies in pleural infection, pneumothorax and malignant pleural effusion, which over the last 15 years have shaped current treatment. He is the co-chair of the BTS Pleural Guidelines 2023, chair of the BTS Pleural Intervention Committee 2023 and chair of multiple ERS guidelines on pleural disease. He was awarded the ERS Mid-Career Gold Medal in Thoracic Oncology in 2021, the ERS Teaching Excellence Award in 2023, and is an NIHR senior investigator.

He is trained in thoracoscopy, thoracic ultrasound and clinical trials methodology. He has published over 200 papers with citations greater than 6,000.

**Radhika Banka** is a Consultant Respiratory Physician at PD Hinduja National Hospital & Medical Research Centre, Mumbai, India. After having completed her respiratory training in India, she moved to the UK where she sub-specialised in the field of pleural medicine at the Oxford Pleural Unit. She has trained in thoracic ultrasound, thoracoscopy and ultrasound-guided pleural procedures. She has a keen interest in thoracic ultrasound and has been on the faculty at various national and international conferences including the BTS and ERS. She was awarded the ERS Silver Sponsorship in 2015 and 2022 to present her research at the ERS Conference. She has published more than 25 papers and was also the sub-editor of the book *Puzzling Cases in Pulmonary Medicine*, published in 2017.

# Contributors

**Dinesh Addala**
NIHR Doctoral Research Fellow
Oxford Pleural Unit and Oxford
    Respiratory Trials Unit
Oxford University
Oxford, UK

**Rachelle Asciak**
Respiratory Consultant
Portsmouth Hospitals University NHS
    Trust
Portsmouth, UK

**Radhika Banka**
Respiratory Consultant
PD Hinduja National Hospital &
    Medical Research Centre
Mumbai, India

**Eihab Bedawi**
Consultant in Respiratory Medicine &
    Pleural Disease
Sheffield Teaching Hospitals NHS
    Foundation Trust

and

Honorary Senior Clinical Lecturer
University of Sheffield
Sheffield, UK

**Poppy Denniston**
Respiratory Registrar
Guy's and St Thomas' Hospital NHS
    Foundation Trust
London, UK

**Mohamed Ellayeh**
Respiratory Consultant
Mansoura University Hospitals
Mansoura, Egypt

**Vineeth George**
Staff Specialist
Department of Respiratory and Sleep
    Medicine
John Hunter Hospital
New Lambton Heights, Australia

**Soumya Ghatak**
Respiratory Registrar
PD Hinduja National Hospital &
    Medical Research Centre
Mumbai, India

**Hui Guo**
Clinical Fellow
Oxford University Hospitals NHS
    Foundation Trust
University of Oxford
Oxford, UK

**Rob Hallifax**
Respiratory Consultant
Oxford University Hospitals NHS
    Foundation Trust

and

Clinical Lecturer
Oxford Respiratory Trials Unit
University of Oxford
Oxford, UK

**Beenish Iqbal**
Pleural Research Fellow
Oxford Respiratory Trials Unit
University of Oxford
Oxford, UK

**Rachel Mercer**
Respiratory Consultant
Portsmouth Hospitals University NHS
    Trust
Portsmouth, UK

**Najib M Rahman**
Professor of Respiratory Medicine and
    Consultant Respiratory Physician
University of Oxford and Oxford
    Centre for Respiratory Medicine
Oxford, UK

**Anand Sundaralingam**
BRC Pleural Research Fellow
Oxford Respiratory Trials Unit
University of Oxford
Oxford, UK

# 1

# A post-operative pleural effusion

## ANAND SUNDARALINGAM

A 70-year-old man was admitted under the surgical team 6 weeks after an elective laparoscopic cholecystectomy. He reported a cough and dyspnoea. The admission chest X-ray (CXR) is shown in Figure 1.1.

a) What is the sensitivity of the CXR for detecting a pleural effusion and how does this compare to CT and ultrasound (US)?

CXR is the least sensitive imaging modality of the three in detecting a pleural effusion. It has been reported that up to 200 ml of fluid would need to accumulate in the pleural space before it would be visible on a postero-anterior (PA) CXR, whereas a smaller volume of 50 ml would be visible on a lateral CXR [1]. In contrast, a US can detect 3–5 ml [2]. In a meta-analysis of 12 studies and 1,554 patients, the pooled sensitivity of US for detecting effusion was 94% (95% CI: 0.88–0.97), whilst CXR was 51% (95% CI: 0.33–0.68) [3]. In practice, a CXR may not always reliably differentiate between pleural effusion and other pathology such as dense consolidation or collapse. For this reason, all pleural interventions for effusions must be conducted under US guidance [4]. CT is an exquisitely sensitive test for the detection of pleural fluid and can detect small pleural effusions, similar to US, although very small effusions can be difficult to differentiate from 'wafer-thin' pleural thickening. In some cases, a prone and supine scan may help differentiate [5].

A right-sided pleural effusion was confirmed on US, and a large volume aspiration (1600 ml) was performed with US guidance (Figure 1.2).

DOI: 10.1201/9781003081630-1

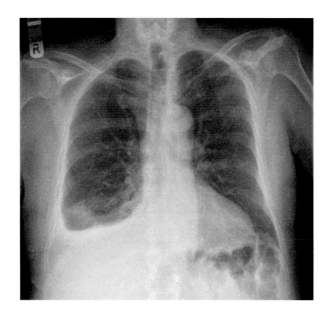

Figure 1.1 CXR on admission with right lower zone opacification.

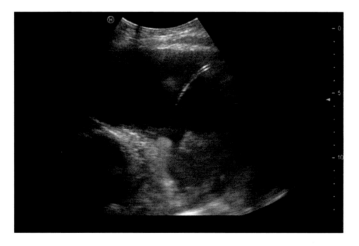

Figure 1.2 TUS image with thoracocentesis catheter in situ.

The pleural fluid returned an exudate: PF (pleural fluid) protein 43 g/L, glucose 7.6 mmol/L, LDH 390 IU/L.

b) What are Light's criteria, their sensitivity and potential drawbacks?

Richard Light's seminal diagnostic criteria for the separation of pleural effusions into transudates and exudates in order to classify the underlying disease state was published in 1972 [6]. His criteria state that observing any one of the following should identify an effusion as an exudate:

- Pleural fluid-to-serum protein ratio >0.5

- Pleural fluid-to-serum LDH ratio >0.6
- Pleural fluid LDH concentration >200 U/L (later changed to two-thirds the upper limit of normal)

Light's criteria are highly sensitive at identifying exudates (99%), however, as a result of such high sensitivity and the need to not miss any potential exudates (that may represent a more serious condition), they can lead to a higher rate of 'false positives', especially when results are close to the aforementioned thresholds. This gives the criteria a reported specificity of 65%–85% and can commonly misclassify transudates as exudates [7].

Further history revealed that the patient had sustained a complicated stay following his surgical procedure, with a large port site bleed, leading to a perihepatic haematoma (Figure 1.3), an intra-operative ventricular tachycardia requiring commencement of amiodarone, on a background of previous myocardial infarction requiring angioplasty 3 years prior to the current admission and post-operative pneumonia.

c) What are your differentials now?

The pleural fluid demonstrates a convincing exudate. This does help narrow the differential list, but it remains extensive, given there are now up to 60 recognised causes of pleural effusion in the literature [8]. The commencement of amiodarone may be of significance; this is a recognised drug-related cause of effusion [9]. However, the commonest cause for an exudative effusion is pleural infection, with an estimated global incidence for empyema of 10–12/100,000 [10].

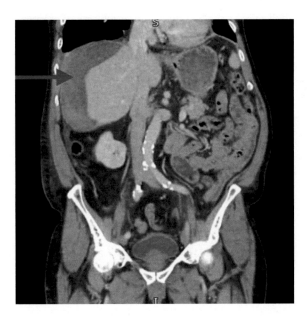

Figure 1.3 CT of the abdomen demonstrating perihepatic haematoma (red arrow).

The effusion was thought to either represent a parapneumonic effusion, drug related or reactive to his post-operative condition. However, it remained recurrent, and he required symptom-guided thoracocentesis on three further occasions, despite cessation of the amiodarone for 8 weeks and radiological resolution of the perihepatic haematoma. When the effusion re-accumulated at 6 months following his initial surgery, an elective thoracoscopy was performed.

d) What is the role of thoracoscopy in undiagnosed pleural effusions?

Local anaesthetic thoracoscopy (LAT) allows direct visual assessment of the pleura and subsequent biopsy of macroscopically abnormal areas. For malignant disease, it has consistently reported diagnostic yields of >90% [11] and similar findings were seen in exudative effusions as a whole [12]. LAT also enables a therapeutic intervention in the same sitting and remains one of the most effective ways of delivering a chemical pleurodesis, with a failure rate of 22% at 3 months [13].

Macroscopically, there was evidence of pleural lymphangitis. Thoracoscopic biopsies revealed dense fibrosis and marked lymphoid infiltrates and were described as showing non-specific pleuritis (Figure 1.4).

e) What is 'non-specific' pleuritis?

Non-specific pleuritis (NSP) describes a constellation of histological findings that are not specific to a single diagnosis, unlike malignant pleuritis, granulomatous pleuritis or pleural vasculitis.

As a result, it may be the histological presentation of many different conditions that leads to an exudative pleural effusion. Several different histological descriptions are used in relation to it. These include reactive fibrous pleural thickening, fibrinous pleurisy, fibrosis, florid reactive change, fibrous

(a)                                    (b)

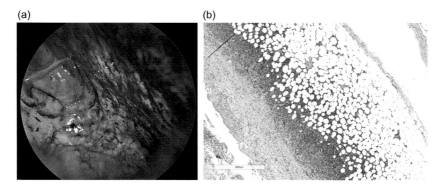

Figure 1.4 (a) Thoracoscopic view of pleural inflammation with vascularisation and hyperaemia, fibrin deposition, and lymphangitic regions. (b) Pleural biopsy histology demonstrating thickened parietal pleura, with inflammatory cell infiltrates.

connective tissue, chronic inflammation, benign change or dense fibrous tissue [14].

Various datasets have described a finding of NSP following pleural biopsy, with a mean incidence of 31%, 95% CI (30%–33%) [14–26]. The pathophysiological mechanisms underpinning NSP are poorly understood, and it may simply represent a final common inflammation or fibrotic pathway.

Given the finding of NSP, the diagnostic net was widened to include a number of rarer conditions. An autoantibody panel revealed only a weakly positive antinuclear antibody (ANA) (1:80) and an IgG4 and amyloid stain on the pleural biopsy returned negative.

f) What are the underlying causes of NSP?

Research and evidence on NSP are largely limited by its retrospective nature.

However, across the existing literature, the underlying aetiology for NSP has been described as:

| | |
|---|---|
| *Idiopathic*: | 48%, 95% CI (45%–50%) [14–21, 23, 25–29] |
| *Pleural infection*: | 15%, 95% CI (13%–18%) [15, 16, 18–20, 23, 26–29] |
| *Benign asbestos related*: | 6%, 95% CI (4%–8%) [14, 15, 18, 23, 27, 30] |
| *Congestive cardiac failure*: | 8%, 95% CI (7%–10%) [15–20, 23, 26, 27, 29, 30] |

It must be noted that retrospective literature describing the aetiology for NSP may simply be describing the underlying disease prevalence for various conditions that give rise to exudative pleural effusions and the differences in clinical practice regarding thoracoscopy across the geographical regions represented in the datasets.

The threshold for describing a case as 'idiopathic' will vary greatly, given there are no standardised definitions for what constitutes an idiopathic cause of NSP. It should only be used following a process of elimination of other possible aetiologies.

Fortunately, the patient's effusion resolved following the thoracoscopy and he required no further pleural interventions. However, given the finding of NSP alongside uncertainty as to the underlying cause, further imaging was arranged at 6-monthly intervals to screen for any evolving malignancies. The CT scan demonstrated resolution of the effusion, however, the patient was left with residual smooth pleural thickening on the right and a new finding of benign-appearing mediastinal lymphadenopathy (Figure 1.5).

g) What is the rate of malignancy following a histological finding of NSP?

Besides the diagnostic uncertainty following a finding of NSP, is whether it represents an accurate result, particularly when the clinical suspicion for a malignant process exists, which is often the case when undertaking a thoracoscopic biopsy. The finding of NSP may represent inadequacies in the biopsy technique, features within the pleural cavity

(a)                                (b)

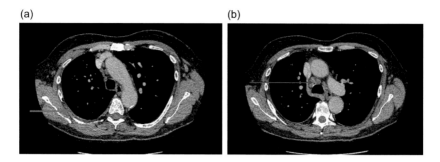

Figure 1.5 (a) Smooth pleural thickening following resolution of pleural effusion (blue arrow). (b) Mediastinal lymphadenopathy (red arrow).

that lead to difficulties in biopsies (e.g. excessive fibrin, adhesions and inadequate views) or it may reflect an early-stage process in the development towards malignancy.

Across existing datasets, malignant transformation occurred in 9%, 95% CI (8%–10%) of cases, with a median time to diagnosis of 6 months (IQR 1–9) [14, 20, 23, 26–31] across a follow-up period ranging from 18 to 64 months [14, 16–18, 20, 21, 23, 25–31]. The majority of cases are malignant pleural mesothelioma.

It is difficult to offer fixed recommendations on the follow-up period for such patients, as it entirely hinges upon the degree of clinical suspicion. Most experts would advocate a 12–24 months follow-up period, with serial imaging at 3–6 monthly intervals, with closer monitoring of those patients in whom there remains a high clinical suspicion, and even pursuing additional methods of biopsy if there is a concern that the thoracoscopic assessment and biopsy were inadequate.

The patient has completed 2 years of interval imaging with respect to the pleural thickening, which has remained stable and is continuing to be monitored for persistent mediastinal lymphadenopathy. To date, he is being managed as a case of NSP and subsequent pleural effusion as a 'reactive' process secondary to his perihepatic haematoma. However, this may yet change in the fullness of time.

## KEY POINTS

- No single test will provide the answer to the cause of a pleural effusion; instead, a combination of history, examination, radiology and pathology is required.
- Observing the behaviour of the pleural effusion over time and the impact of trials of therapy can be powerful tools to differentiate between aetiologies.
- NSP is a broad histological definition and encompasses many different causes of an exudative pleural effusion.

- Following a result of NSP, clinicians must assess how likely this represents a true result and base their subsequent investigation and monitoring plan on this assessment, bearing in mind that approximately 9% of cases will progress to pleural malignancy.

## REFERENCES

1. Blackmore CC, Black WC, Dallas RV, Crow HC. Pleural fluid volume estimation: A chest radiograph prediction rule. *Acad Radiol.* 1996;3(2):103–109.
2. Gryminski J, Krakówka P, Lypacewicz G. The diagnosis of pleural effusion by ultrasonic and radiologic techniques. *Chest.* 1976;70(1):33–37.
3. Yousefifard M, Baikpour M, Ghelichkhani P, Asady H, Shahsavari Nia K, Moghadas Jafari A, Hosseini M, Safari S. Screening performance characteristic of ultrasonography and radiography in detection of pleural effusion; a meta-analysis. *Emergency.* 2016;4(1):1–10.
4. Havelock T, Teoh R, Laws D, Gleeson F, BTS Pleural Disease Guideline Group. Pleural procedures and thoracic ultrasound: British Thoracic Society pleural disease guideline 2010. *Thorax.* 2010;65(Supp 2):ii61–ii76.
5. Duerden L, Benamore R, Edey A. Radiology: What is the role of chest radiographs, CT and PET in modern management? In CB Maskell, NA Laursen, Lee YCG, Rahman NM eds. *Pleural Disease European Respiratory Society Monograph.* European Respiratory Society, Sheffield; 2020. pp. 48–72.
6. Light RW, Macgregor MI, Luchsinger PC, Ball WC. Pleural effusions: The diagnostic separation of transudates and exudates. *Ann Intern Med.* 1972;77(4):507–513.
7. Heffner JE. Discriminating between transudates and exudates. *Clin Chest Med.* 2006;27(2):241–252.
8. Feller-Kopman D, Light R. Pleural disease. *N Engl J Med.* 2018;378(8): 740–751.
9. Hooper C, Lee GYC, Maskell NA, BTS Pleural Disease Guideline Group. Investigation of a unilateral pleural effusion in adults: British Thoracic Society pleural disease guideline 2010. *Thorax.* 2010;65(Supp 2):ii4–ii17.
10. Bodtger U, Hallifax RJ. Epidemiology: Why is pleural disease becoming more common? In CB Maskell, NA Laursen, Lee YCG, Rahman NM eds. *Pleural Disease European Respiratory Society Monograph.* European Respiratory Society, Sheffield. 2020; pp. 1–12.
11. Rahman NM, Ali N, Brown G, Chapman S, Davies RJO, Gleeson FV, Howes TQ, Treasure T, Singh S, Philips G, BTS Pleural Disease Guideline Group. Local anaesthetic thoracoscopy: British Thoracic Society pleural disease guideline 2010. *Thorax.* 2010;65(Supp 2):ii54–ii60.
12. Agarwal R, Aggarwal AN, Gupta D. Diagnostic accuracy and safety of semirigid thoracoscopy in exudative pleural effusions: A meta-analysis. *Chest.* 2013;144(6):1857–1867.

13. Bhatnagar R, Piotrowska HEG, Laskawiec-Szkonter M, et al. Effect of thoracoscopic talc poudrage vs talc slurry via chest tube on pleurodesis failure rate among patients with malignant pleural effusions: A randomized clinical trial. *JAMA - J Am Med Assoc.* 2020;323(1):60–69.

14. Davies HE, Nicholson JE, Rahman NM, Wilkinson EM, Davies RJO, Lee YCG. Outcome of patients with nonspecific pleuritis/fibrosis on thoracoscopic pleural biopsies. *Eur J Cardio-Thorac Surg.* 2010;38(4):472–477.

15. Boutin C, Viallat JR, Cargnino P, Farisse P. Thoracoscopy in malignant pleural effusions. *Am Rev Respir Dis.* 1981;124(5):588–592.

16. Page RD, Jeffrey RR, Donnelly RJ. Thoracoscopy: A review of 121 consecutive surgical procedures. *Ann Thorac Surg.* 1989;48(1):66–68.

17. Hucker J, Bhatnagar NK, al-Jilaihawi AN, Forrester-Wood CP. Thoracoscopy in the diagnosis and management of recurrent pleural effusions. *Ann Thorac Surg.* 1991;52(5):1145–1147.

18. Menzies R, Charbonneau M. Thoracoscopy for the diagnosis of pleural disease. *Ann Intern Med.* 1991;114(4):271–276.

19. Ohri SK, Oswal SK, Townsend ER, Fountain SW. Early and late outcome after diagnostic thoracoscopy and talc pleurodesis. *Ann Thorac Surg.* 1992;53(6):1038–1041.

20. Kendall SW, Bryan AJ, Large SR, Wells FC. Pleural effusions: Is thoracoscopy a reliable investigation? A retrospective review. *Respir Med.* 1992;86(5):437–440.

21. Hansen M, Faurschou P, Clementsen P. Medical thoracoscopy, results and complications in 146 patients: A retrospective study. *Respir Med.* 1998;92(2):228–232.

22. Blanc F-X, Atassi K, Bignon J, Housset B. Diagnostic value of medical thoracoscopy in pleural disease: A 6-year retrospective study. *Chest.* 2002;121(5):1677–1683.

23. Janssen JP, Ramlal S, Mravunac M. The long-term follow up of exudative pleural effusion after nondiagnostic thoracoscopy. *J Bronchol.* 2004;11(3):169–174.

24. Metintas MG, Cadirci O, Yildirim H, Dundar E, Metintas S. Outcome of patients diagnosed with fibrinous pleuritis after medical thoracoscopy. *Respir Med.* 2012;106(8):1177–1183.

25. Vakil E, Ost D, Vial MR, Stewart J, Sarkiss MG, Morice RC, Casal RF, Eapen GA, Grosu HB. Non-specific pleuritis in patients with active malignancy. *Respirol Carlton Vic.* 2018;23(2):213–219.

26. Yu Y-X, Yang Y, Wu Y-B, Wang X-J, Xu L-L, Wang Z, Wang F, Tong Z-H, Shi H-Z. An update of the long-term outcome of patients with nonspecific pleurisy at medical thoracoscopy. *BMC Pulm Med.* 2021;21(1):226.

27. Venekamp LN, Velkeniers B, Noppen M. Does "idiopathic pleuritis" exist? Natural history of non-specific pleuritis diagnosed after thoracoscopy. *Respir Int Rev Thorac Dis.* 2005;72(1):74–78.

28. DePew ZS, Verma A, Wigle D, Mullon JJ, Nichols FC, Maldonado F. Nonspecific pleuritis: Optimal duration of follow-up. *Ann Thorac Surg.* 2014;97(6):1867–1871.

29. Gunluoglu G, Olcmen A, Gunluoglu MZ, Dincer I, Sayar A, Camsari G, Yilmaz V, Altin S. Long-term outcome of patients with undiagnosed pleural effusion. *Arch Bronconeumol.* 2015;51(12):632–636.

30. Ferrer JS, Muñoz XG, Orriols RM, Light RW, Morell FB. Evolution of idiopathic pleural effusion: A prospective, long-term follow-up study. *Chest.* 1996;109(6):1508–1513.

31. Karpathiou G, Anevlavis S, Tiffet O, et al. Clinical long-term outcome of non-specific pleuritis (NSP) after surgical or medical thoracoscopy. *J Thorac Dis.* 2020;12(5):2096–2104.

# 2

# Pleural effusion and chest pain in an elderly gentleman

## MOHAMED ELLAYEH

A 79-year-old man presented to the respiratory service in 2019 with intermittent dull right-sided chest pain and breathlessness. He was an ex-smoker of 20 years, and worked in coal mines, engineering and machine repair. The presenting chest X-ray demonstrated well-defined right-upper and middle-lobe peripheral opacification with an associated moderate right-sided pleural effusion.

a) What is the incidence and presentation of malignant pleural effusion?

Malignant pleural effusion (MPE) is a condition affecting thousands of patients per year in Europe and the USA. The most common causes of MPE include secondary spread from lung and breast cancer, and lymphoma. The median survival time averages between 3 and 12 months. Pleural malignancy is associated with high hospital admissions, costs and mortality (1). Although there have been major advances in the treatment of cancer, in MPE treatment is directed towards palliation of symptoms and improving quality of life (2).

Dyspnoea is the most frequent initial presenting symptom, followed by cough, chest pain, non-specific fatigue and loss of weight. Dyspnoea may be disproportionate to the amount of effusion at presentation. Patients with MPE may present with paraneoplastic syndromes such as inappropriate secretion of anti-diuretic hormone, or haematologic, neurologic or renal diseases (3).

The patient complained of intermittent right-sided dull chest pain and breathlessness for the last month, with no apparent trigger. Two weeks before presentation,

DOI: 10.1201/9781003081630-2

his partner noticed a deterioration in his exercise tolerance. He now developed breathlessness on walking more than five stairs and was sleeping on three pillows, accompanied by loss of appetite and weight.

After drainage of the pleural effusion, breathlessness improved significantly, and he was able to walk more easily with a performance status of 1.

b) What is the role of imaging in the diagnosis of malignant pleural effusion?

Chest X-ray: The presentation is mostly unilateral with only 5% of cases presenting with bilateral effusions. Patients with a history of asbestos exposure may have pleural plaques (calcified or non-calcified).

Ultrasound (US): The presence of pleural nodularity on the costoparietal, visceral and/or diaphragmatic pleural surfaces can be indicative of malignancy, as is the presence of parietal thickening >1 cm, diaphragm thickness of >7 mm or inability to resolve the normal layers of the diaphragm.

CT: Characteristic features of malignancy includes nodularity, circumferential thickened pleura, mediastinal pleural involvement and parietal pleural thickening of more than 1 cm.

PET/CT: Can be used to assess the metastatic spread, in addition to a slightly higher sensitivity for malignant diagnosis (4), but this does not exceed around 80%.

The chest X-ray showed a well-defined, large, right-upper and middle-zone peripheral opacification. There was associated blunting of the right costophrenic angle (Figure 2.1). Thoracic US showed a grossly abnormal para-diaphragmatic mass of 6 cm depth in association with a large effusion (Figure 2.2). A thoracic CT scan showed a moderate right pleural effusion with associated malignant pleural thickening. There were subtle bilateral partly calcified pleural plaques with a 6 cm smoothly marginated, heterogeneously enhancing mass in the periphery of the right-upper lobe, which invaded the chest wall, extending into the extrapleural fat. There was no associated bone destruction (Figure 2.3).

c) What are the methods for diagnosing MPE?

The first step in establishing a diagnosis of MPE is cytology. Cytology has a diagnostic accuracy of 60%, with extremely poor sensitivity for mesothelioma (6%) and higher sensitivity for adenocarcinomas (79%). Immunohistochemistry, which exposes reactive mesothelial cells to distinct antibody panels, can help differentiate malignant pleural mesothelioma and adenocarcinoma. The gold standard technique for diagnosing MPE is a pleural biopsy. Percutaneous non-image-guided pleural biopsy has a poorer diagnostic sensitivity (46%) when compared to image guided techniques, with sensitivity increasing to up to 90% when the biopsy is guided by US or CT. The diagnostic

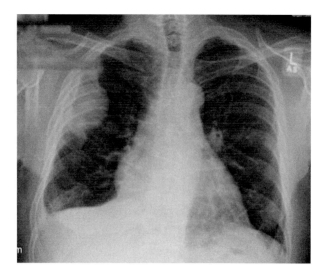

Figure 2.1 Chest X-ray showing well-defined, large, right-upper and middle-zone peripheral opacification. There is associated blunting of the right costo-phrenic angle.

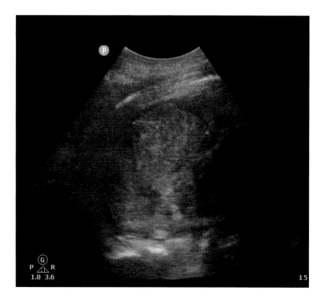

Figure 2.2 Ultrasound image of right thorax showing large pleural-based mass.

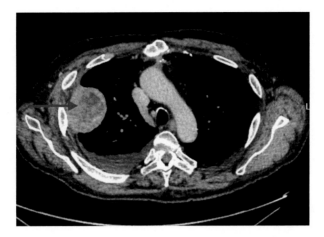

Figure 2.3 Mediastinal window of CT thorax showing right heterogenous pleural mass (arrow) with pleural effusion.

sensitivity of CT-guided biopsy in MPE is comparable to that of thoracoscopy (96% vs 95%), especially when the pleural thickening is more than 1 cm. Pleural biopsy can be conducted via thoracoscopy (medical thoracoscopy or video-assisted thoracoscopic surgery [VATS]) when the pleural thickening is not visible on ultrasound, or when it is difficult to access. Both techniques are valuable to concurrently visualise the pleura, take a biopsy from the affected areas, drain pleural fluid and conduct pleurodesis in one sitting. Medical thoracoscopy is a safe technique with minimal rates of complications and a good diagnostic yield. It is effective in patients with contraindications for surgery or patients who cannot tolerate general anaesthesia in VATS (5).

Cytology from two different samples of pleural fluid showed neutrophil-rich fluid, with no malignant cells. Thoracoscopy was conducted and macroscopic evaluation showed few pleural plaques and some areas of pleural inflammation. The apical lobe was adhered to the chest wall and therefore the pleural above was not examined, but there were some areas of subtle pleural nodularity, highly suggestive of malignant disease. A large vascular and anterior pleural mass adjacent to diaphragmatic pleura was identified (Figures 2.4 and 2.5).

Histopathological examination showed a malignant spindle cell tumour consistent with sarcomatoid mesothelioma.

d) When should pleurodesis be performed in malignant pleural effusion?

Recurring MPEs were originally managed with chest catheter placement followed by chemical pleurodesis as a first-line treatment, with indwelling pleural catheter (IPC) placement reserved for patients who had a trapped lung or pleurodesis failure. There has been a recent trend toward considering IPC as a suitable first-line alternative option to talc pleurodesis, with

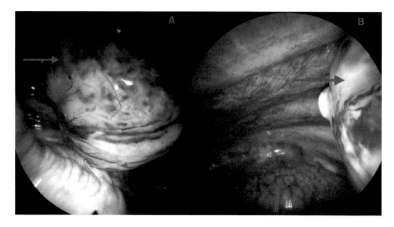

Figure 2.4 (A and B) Thoracoscopic image showing vascular mass adjacent to the diaphragm (arrow).

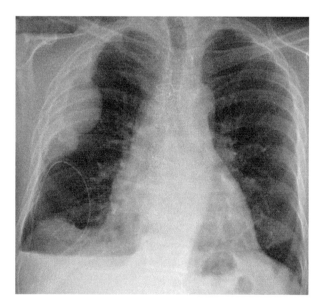

Figure 2.5 Chest X-ray after insertion of indwelling pleural catheter on the right hemithorax.

randomised evidence demonstrating no difference in symptom relief between the two techniques (6, 7). Talc (graded) is considered to be the intrapleural pleurodesis agent of choice, as it is highly effective and safe. After instillation in the pleural space, an inflammatory reaction occurs. This reaction leads to the adhesion of the pleural surfaces and obliteration of the pleural space. The most frequent adverse effects of talc pleurodesis are pain

(7%), fever (mostly low grade), infection at the catheter site and empyema (rare). Acute respiratory distress syndrome with some evidence of mortality in around 4% of patients has been noted with non-graded talc.

Successful pleurodesis includes two categories: (1) complete success, which refers to the longstanding absence of symptoms caused by malignant effusion, with lack of fluid recurrence on radiology till death; and (2) partial success, which refers to decreased breathlessness caused by effusion, with only partial fluid recurrence with no additional therapeutic aspirations needed. Trapped lung increases the likelihood of talc pleurodesis failure and these patients are best managed by IPC placement (8).

On follow-up 2 weeks after thoracoscopy, the patient complained of breathlessness. Pleural ultrasound showed an echogenic pleural effusion with a maximum depth of 6 cm in the craniocaudal plane of over three rib spaces. An IPC was placed to alleviate the breathlessness after discussion of the available treatment options with the patient (Figure 2.6).

e) What are the management options for mesothelioma?

According to the patient's preference, talc (slurry or poudrage) or IPC is offered for management of symptomatic effusion. Talc (slurry or poudrage) is preferable in the management of symptomatic effusion when compared to video-assisted thoracoscopic surgery partial pleurectomy (VATSPP), as demonstrated by a randomised trial which showed that there was no survival benefit for surgical approaches compared to physician-delivered talc

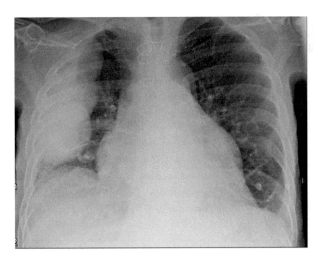

Figure 2.6 Chest X-ray showing the increase in pleural-based mass during follow-up.

in mesothelioma, and increased costs and complications (9). Cisplatin and pemetrexed are recommended as first-line therapy in patients with good performance status, and recent evidence has suggested that combined immunotherapy (nivolumab and ipilimumab) is potentially more effective, especially in non-epithelioid subtypes (10). In addition, randomised data suggests bevacizumab in addition to standard chemotherapy prolongs survival, but this is not widely available and does have some side effects. Prophylactic radiation, and pre-operative and post-operative radiotherapy are not recommended in the management of mesothelioma, based on a randomised trial demonstrating no benefit (11). However, patients should be carefully monitored for the complication of catheter tract metastasis. Furthermore, it is recommended to refer mesothelioma cases to a regional multidisciplinary team (10).

The case was staged as T4N1M0 (due to chest wall invasion and mediastinal node involvement), and histopathology was consistent with sarcomatoid/biphasic mesothelioma. An IPC was inserted for pleural fluid control according to patient choice. Treatment with combination immunotherapy (ipilimumab and nivolumab) was started. After two cycles, he presented with neutropenic sepsis and empyema, which responded to antibiotics and drainage. Follow-up imaging showed an increase in the size of the pleural-based mass, which made the likelihood of benefit from further chemotherapy very low, in addition to a decline in performance status. A decision was made to stop chemotherapy and to direct the management plan to increase his quality of life through supportive care.

## KEY POINTS

- Mesothelioma is a relatively uncommon diagnosis (depending on prevalence) but should be considered, especially in cytology-negative exudates in asbestos-exposed individuals.
- Diagnosis usually requires a biopsy with a high level of cytology-negative samples.
- Treatment for mesothelioma focuses on symptom management (especially of pleural fluid, which tends to be recurrent) and then systemic anti-cancer therapy, which should be managed by an oncologist with experience in mesothelioma management.

## REFERENCES

1. Mummadi SR, Stoller JK, Lopez R, Kailasam K, Gillespie CT, Hahn PY. Epidemiology of adult pleural disease in the United States. *Chest.* 2021;160(4):1534–1551.
2. Bedawi EO, Guinde J, Rahman NM, Astoul P. Advances in pleural infection and malignancy. *Eur Respir Rev.* 2021;30(159):200002.
3. Kastelik JA. Management of malignant pleural effusion. *Lung.* 2013;191(2):165–175.

4. Hallifax RJ, Talwar A, Wrightson JM, Edey A, Gleeson FV. State-of-the-art: Radiological investigation of pleural disease. *Respir Med.* 2017;124:88–99.

5. Ferreiro L, Suárez-Antelo J, Álvarez-Dobaño JM, Toubes ME, Riveiro V, Valdés L. Malignant pleural effusion: Diagnosis and management. *Can Respir J.* 2020;2020:2950751.

6. Davies HE, Mishra EK, Kahan BC, et al. Effect of an indwelling pleural catheter vs chest tube and talc pleurodesis for relieving dyspnea in patients with malignant pleural effusion: The TIME2 randomized controlled trial. *JAMA.* 2012;307(22):2383–2389.

7. Thomas R, Fysh ETH, Smith NA, et al. Effect of an indwelling pleural catheter vs talc pleurodesis on hospitalization days in patients with malignant pleural effusion: The AMPLE randomized clinical trial. *JAMA.* 2017;318(19):1903–1912.

8. Asciak R, Rahman NM. Malignant pleural effusion: From diagnostics to therapeutics. *Clin Chest Med.* 2018;39(1):181–193.

9. Rintoul RC, Ritchie AJ, Edwards JG, et al. Efficacy and cost of video-assisted thoracoscopic partial pleurectomy versus talc pleurodesis in patients with malignant pleural mesothelioma (MesoVATS): An open-label, randomised, controlled trial. *Lancet.* 2014;384(9948):1118–1127.

10. Woolhouse I, Maskell NA. Introducing the new BTS guideline: The investigation and management of pleural malignant mesothelioma. *Thorax.* 2018;73(3):210–212.

11. Clive AO, Taylor H, Dobson L, et al. Prophylactic radiotherapy for the prevention of procedure-tract metastases after surgical and large-bore pleural procedures in malignant pleural mesothelioma (SMART): A multicentre, open-label, phase 3, randomised controlled trial. *Lancet Oncol.* 2016;17(8):1094–1104.

# 3

# A difficult-to-drain effusion

VINEETH GEORGE

A 75-year-old gentleman was referred to the pleural service with a subacute history of weight loss and progressive dyspnoea in the context of occupational asbestos exposure. Thoracic ultrasound demonstrated a moderate echogenic effusion with nodular pleural thickening. He underwent thoracocentesis, which was cytology negative. He was considered unfit for thoracoscopy due to performance status, and an ultrasound-guided pleural biopsy was performed which confirmed a diagnosis of epithelioid mesothelioma.

a) How is a septated malignant pleural effusion (MPE) diagnosed?

Septations, which are fibrinous strands within pleural fluid, are caused by pleural inflammation (1). They can be seen in exudative conditions of any cause but are frequently seen in malignant pleural effusions (2). Their presence can limit the drainage of effusions, and the number of septations seen on ultrasound is negatively correlated with post-procedural improvement in dyspnoea (3).

Data from pleural infection cohorts demonstrate that ultrasound is superior to CT in the detection of septations, and septations are increasingly being identified as the use of ultrasound becomes more widespread (4, 5). This is also supported by studies of individuals undergoing thoracic surgery, which suggest that pleural adhesions, which are generally considered to be denser, are also better seen on ultrasound. A study of 64 consecutive patients undergoing video-assisted thoracoscopic surgery (VATS), CT reported a sensitivity of 71% and a specificity of 72% for diagnosis of septations (6). In contrast, patients undergoing thoracic ultrasound prior to surgery have reported sensitivities of 81%–88% with specificity of 83%–96% (7, 8).

The degree of septation on ultrasound can also be quantified with an objective septation score based on the maximum number of septations in a single ultrasound field. This septation score on pre-procedural ultrasound

DOI: 10.1201/9781003081630-3

is inversely correlated with symptomatic relief from pleural effusion drainage (3).

Septations are also frequently seen directly at thoracoscopy, with one large retrospective analysis reporting that they were seen to some degree in 60% of patients undergoing local anaesthetic thoracoscopy (2).

Patients with non-draining septated MPEs have higher pleural fluid lactate dehydrogenase (LDH) and serum C-reactive protein (CRP) levels than unselected patients with MPE (9), although at this stage there is no evidence to support the use of serum markers to detect septations in MPE.

On review in clinic, he reported ongoing breathlessness and his effusion was found to be moderately septated (Figure 3.1). An indwelling pleural catheter (IPC) was inserted a week later to provide definitive control of dyspnoea.

b) What is the role of IPCs in septated MPE?

Heavily septated effusions are less likely to drain completely and pleural apposition is less likely to be achieved (10). Consequently, patients with heavy septations have been considered unsuitable for traditional pleurodesis, with IPCs increasingly used in this setting (10). However, there is limited high-quality data supporting this approach.

IPC-related symptomatic loculations can also develop in up to 14% of patients with IPCs (11). This is thought to be secondary to fibrin deposition, either due to the IPC itself or from associated inflammation. Despite its frequent occurrence, data to guide management in this setting is limited to small retrospective case series.

The largest of these, by Vial and colleagues, identified 97 patients with a non-draining IPC and a persistent pleural effusion who were treated with tissue plasminogen activator (tPA) (12). Of these, 79 (81%) had some degree

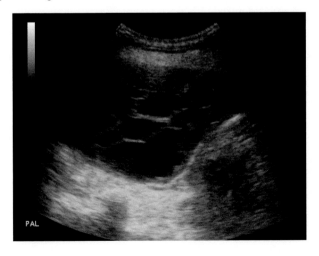

Figure 3.1 Ultrasound image of a moderately septated effusion.

of loculation. Drainage was restored in 83 out of 97 patients (86%, 95% CI 77%–92%) after one dose of tPA.

Similarly, Thomas et al. reported that pleural fluid drainage improved in 93% of patients, with dyspnoea improving in 83%, who received fibrinolytics for symptomatic IPC-related loculation (13). The majority of these instillations were performed in the outpatient setting (61%). A variety of fibrinolytic agents were used, with tPA being used most frequently (n = 52, 79%) (13). However, the response to treatment was often not durable with 41% of patients experiencing a recurrence of symptomatic loculations at a median of 13 days, with only one patient of the ten who received a second dose having a sustained improvement in drainage and symptoms.

The risk of bleeding across these two series was low with a total of four cases of non-fatal bleeding encountered out of the 163 patients (2%) (12, 13).

Approximately 4 weeks after insertion, the IPC drainage slowed dramatically and he re-presented to the pleural service for review. There were no new systemic symptoms. The catheter flushed adequately, but thoracic ultrasound demonstrated that the effusion was now heavily septated (Figure 3.2).

c) How do you differentiate between malignancy and infection in septated effusions?

Septations can occur with exudative effusions of any cause but are most associated with MPE or pleural infection (14).

Differentiating pleural infection from MPE, particularly in the context of cytology-negative inflammatory malignancy, can be difficult and one needs to consider the overall clinical picture. Single-centre, retrospective data suggest that patients presenting with MPE are frequently prescribed antibiotics

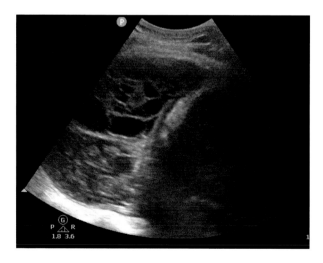

Figure 3.2 Ultrasound image of a heavily septated effusion.

and that the ability to promptly and accurately differentiate malignancy from infection is poor even in the tertiary setting (15).

Routinely used serum and pleural biomarkers such as CRP and pleural fluid glucose are non-specific markers of inflammation (16, 17). Of these, serum procalcitonin has been reported to be a marker for bacterial sepsis in a number of settings (18). However, data supporting its use to discriminate between pleural infection and other aetiologies, such as MPE, has been conflicting (16, 17).

Data from the AUDIO (Advanced Ultrasound in Pleural Infection) study, which was a 20-patient pilot study, has suggested that ultrasound-guided pleural biopsy can increase microbiological yield in pleural infection (19). This adds to data demonstrating that physician-delivered, ultrasound-guided pleural biopsy is safe and has a high sensitivity for diagnosing MPE (20). Further studies to evaluate the routine use of this technique in undifferentiated effusion are needed.

Intrapleural alteplase was trialled via the IPC, which resulted in increased drainage volumes and reduced breathlessness. This was instilled on two more occasions over 6 months with good symptomatic effect but with no change in the underlying performance status.

d) What is the role of intrapleural fibrinolytic therapy in MPE?

The use of intrapleural fibrinolytics for septated malignant pleural effusions developed after extrapolation from its successful use in the setting of pleural infection (13, 21). Ultrasound imaging has shown that intrapleural fibrinolytics can lyse pleural septations (22).

To date, three randomised controlled trials have evaluated the efficacy of intrapleural fibrinolytics with standard chest tubes (5). However, none have shown that intrapleural fibrinolytic therapy improves clinically significant outcome measures. The largest of these, the TIME 3 trial, was a double-blind, placebo-controlled trial which randomised 71 patients with a non-draining malignant pleural effusion to intrapleural urokinase versus placebo (23). Although the urokinase group demonstrated significant improvement in a range of secondary outcomes including radiological appearance, length of stay and survival, there was no significant difference in the two co-primary outcome measures of the trial: dyspnoea change as measured on a 100 mm VAS scale or pleurodesis success.

This study demonstrates that radiological improvement does not necessarily translate to improved breathlessness for patients with septated MPE. It also suggests that intrapleural fibrinolytics should not be routinely used for this patient population. However, the unexpectedly poor survival in this trial (with a median survival of 48 days in the placebo group) raises the possibility that selected patients with a more robust prognosis may still benefit from fibrinolytic therapy.

Unfortunately, his overall health declined further and after discussion with the patient and family, it was thought that further pleural intervention would not be of benefit. He was managed with non-interventional measures to control dyspnoea and passed away peacefully 15 months after the initial diagnosis.

## KEY POINTS

- Septations are frequently seen in malignant pleural effusion and are best diagnosed on thoracic ultrasound.
- Complete drainage and pleural apposition can be difficult to achieve in the context of heavy septation, and IPCs are increasingly used for this subgroup of patients.
- Differentiating infection from malignancy can be difficult in this setting, and assessing the clinical context is vital.
- Therapeutic options are limited for patients with septated MPE, but intrapleural fibrinolytic therapy may be of benefit in selected cases.

## REFERENCES

1. Bibby AC, Dorn P, Psallidas I, Porcel JM, Janssen J, Froudarakis M, et al. ERS/EACTS statement on the management of malignant pleural effusions. *The European Respiratory Journal*. 2018 July;52(1):1800349.
2. Bielsa S, Martín-Juan J, Porcel JM, Rodríguez-Panadero F. Diagnostic and prognostic implications of pleural adhesions in malignant effusions. *Journal of Thoracic Oncology*. 2008;3(11):1251–6.
3. Psallidas I, Yousuf A, Talwar A, Hallifax RJ, Mishra EK, Corcoran JP, et al. Assessment of patient-reported outcome measures in pleural interventions. *BMJ Open Respiratory Research*. 2017 July 1;4(1):e000171.
4. Porcel JM. Chest imaging for the diagnosis of complicated parapneumonic effusions. Vol. 24, *Current Opinion in Pulmonary Medicine*. Lippincott Williams and Wilkins; 2018. pp. 398–402.
5. Banka R, Terrington D, Mishra EK. Management of septated malignant pleural effusions. *Current Pulmonology Reports*. 2018 February;7(1):1–5.
6. Mason AC, Miller BH, Krasna MJ, White CS. Accuracy of CT for the detection of pleural adhesions: Correlation with video-assisted thoracoscopic surgery. *Chest*. 1999 February;115(2):423–7.
7. Cassanelli N, Caroli G, Dolci G, Dell'amore A, Luciano G, Bini A, et al. Accuracy of transthoracic ultrasound for the detection of pleural adhesions. *European Journal of Cardio-Thoracic Surgery*. 2012 November;42(5):813–8.
8. Wei B, Wang T, Jiang F, Wang H. Use of transthoracic ultrasound to predict pleural adhesions: A prospective blinded study. *The Thoracic and Cardiovascular Surgeon*. 2012 March 25;60(02):101–4.

9. Mishra E, Clive A, Davies H, Nunn A, Miller R, Psallidas I, et al. P234 Patient and fluid characteristics associated with non-draining malignant pleural effusion. In: *Closing the Flood Gates of the Pleura*. BMJ Publishing Group Ltd and British Thoracic Society; 2017. pp. A210.2–A211.

10. Walker S, Bibby AC, Maskell NA. Current best practice in the evaluation and management of malignant pleural effusions. Vol. 11, *Therapeutic Advances in Respiratory Disease*. SAGE Publications Ltd; 2017. pp. 105–14.

11. Fysh ETH, Waterer GW, Kendall PA, Bremner PR, Dina S, Geelhoed E, et al. Indwelling pleural catheters reduce inpatient days over pleurodesis for malignant pleural effusion. *Chest*. 2012;142(2):394–400.

12. Vial MR, Ost DE, Eapen GA, Jimenez CA, Morice RC, O'Connell O, et al. Intrapleural fibrinolytic therapy in patients with nondraining indwelling pleural catheters. *Journal of Bronchology and Interventional Pulmonology*. 2016;23(2):98–105.

13. Thomas R, Piccolo F, Miller D, MacEachern PR, Chee AC, Huseini T, et al. Intrapleural fibrinolysis for the treatment of indwelling pleural catheter-related symptomatic loculations: A multicenter observational study. *Chest*. 2015 September 1;148(3):746–51.

14. Hallifax RJ, Talwar A, Wrightson JM, Edey A, Gleeson FV. State-of-the-art: Radiological investigation of pleural disease. *Respiratory Medicine*. 2017;124:88–99.

15. George V, Mercer R, Bedawi E, Dudina A, Rahman N. P103 Antibiotic use and comorbid pleural infection in patients with malignant pleural effusion. *Thorax*. 2019 December 1;74(Suppl 2):A146 LP-A147.

16. Dixon G, Lama-Lopez A, Bintcliffe OJ, Morley AJ, Hooper CE, Maskell NA. The role of serum procalcitonin in establishing the diagnosis and prognosis of pleural infection. *Respiratory Research*. 2017 February;18(1):30.

17. McCann FJ, Chapman SJ, Yu WC, Maskell NA, Davies RJO, Lee YCG. Ability of procalcitonin to discriminate infection from non-infective inflammation using two pleural disease settings. *PLOS ONE*. 2012;7(12).

18. Creamer AW, Kent AE, Albur M. Procalcitonin in respiratory disease: Use as a biomarker for diagnosis and guiding antibiotic therapy. *Breathe*. 2019;15(4):296–304.

19. Psallidas I, Kanellakis NI, Bhatnagar R, Ravindran R, Yousuf A, Edey AJ, et al. A pilot feasibility study in establishing the role of ultrasound-guided pleural biopsies in pleural infection (the AUDIO study). *Chest*. 2018;154(4):766–72.

20. Hallifax RJ, Corcoran JP, Ahmed A, Nagendran M, Rostom H, Hassan N, et al. Physician-based ultrasound-guided biopsy for diagnosing pleural disease. *Chest*. 2014;146(4):1001–6.

21. Rahman NM, Maskell NA, West A, Teoh R, Arnold A, Mackinlay C, et al. Intrapleural use of tissue plasminogen activator and DNase in pleural infection. *New England Journal of Medicine.* 2011;365(6):518–26.
22. Maskell NA, Gleeson FV. Images in clinical medicine. Effect of intrapleural streptokinase on a loculated malignant pleural effusion. *New England Journal of Medicine.* 2003;348(14):e4.
23. Mishra EK, Clive AO, Wills GH, Davies HE, Stanton AE, Al-Aloul M, et al. Randomized controlled trial of urokinase versus placebo for nondraining malignant pleural effusion. *American Journal of Respiratory and Critical Care Medicine.* 2018;197:502–8.

# 4

# A recurrent and persistent effusion

EIHAB BEDAWI

A 74-year-old retired carpenter was referred with a 'pleural abnormality' incidentally found on CT for investigation of a bladder tumour. He was an ex-smoker with moderate COPD, heart failure with midrange ejection fraction (HF-mREF), rheumatoid arthritis (RA; quiescent on methotrexate), low-grade bladder tumour (under surveillance) and factor VII deficiency. He had a performance status of 1 and was asymptomatic.

a) What do the CT images in Figure 4.1 show and what is the best course of action based on these findings?

The CT shows left-sided pleural thickening with evidence of pleural plaques (yellow arrow) in keeping with previous asbestos exposure. There are no features of malignant pleural disease (as described in Chapter 2). The thickening is smooth with evidence of rounded atelectasis (blue arrow) and extrapleural fat hypertrophy (red arrow). Pleural plaques alone do not require radiological follow-up, but in the presence of thickening and asbestos exposure, CT follow-up for 2 years would be a reasonable course of action based on data from studies looking at the likelihood of non-specific pleuritis progressing to pleural malignancy (1, 2).

He was followed up radiologically for 2 years with no evidence of progression and discharged. Two years later, he presented with exertional breathlessness over 2 months that had become acutely worse over days. He had right pleuritic chest pain but no cough, fevers, weight loss or night sweats, and his appetite had been stable. A chest X-ray showed evidence of a large, right-sided loculated pleural effusion and he went on to have a CT scan (Figure 4.2). A CT urogram showed no evidence of recurrence of bladder cancer.

DOI: 10.1201/9781003081630-4

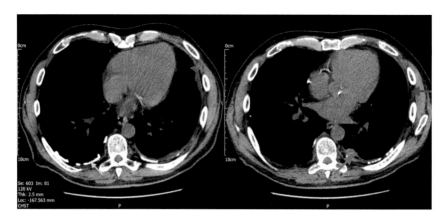

Figure 4.1 Mediastinal window of thoracic CT showing the presence of pleural plaques (yellow arrow), rounded atelectasis (blue arrow) and extrapleural fat hypertrophy (red arrow).

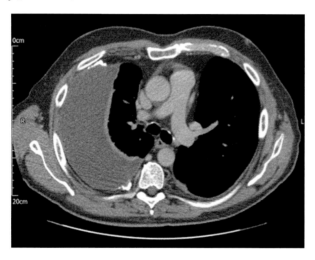

Figure 4.2 Mediastinal window of thoracic CT showing the presence of a large, right-sided pleural effusion with underlying pleural enhancement.

*Bloods* – WCC 5900/mm³, platelets 302000/mm³, CRP 9.2 mg/L, albumin
  31 g/L, urea 3.8 mmol/L
*PF biochemistry* – pH 7.32, protein 47 g/dL, glucose 2.8 mmol/L, LDH 854 IU/L
*PF microscopy and culture* – negative
*PF cytology* – heavily bloodstained fluid, inflammatory cells only

Given the suspicion of malignancy (either mesothelioma or pleural malignancy secondary to urological primary), a medical thoracoscopy was conducted. Macroscopically, this showed diffuse pleural thickening and inflammation but no visible pleural or diaphragmatic nodularity. Several pleural strip biopsies were taken down to fat and an indwelling pleural catheter (IPC) was inserted for definitive fluid control following pre-discussion with the patient. The histopathology review confirmed no evidence of malignancy and demonstrated fibrosis only.

b) What is the most likely diagnosis so far?

This patient has features of rheumatoid pleuritis. Pleural involvement in RA is common with autopsy studies ranging from 40% to 75%, but only 5%–20% of patients complain of pleurisy and just over 5% have a radiological effusion. It occurs predominantly in males, and chest pain (± fever) is the most common symptom. Pleural fluid typically contains low WCC, low glucose and a moderately elevated LDH (>700 IU/L). Chronic pleural inflammation can cause chylous effusions, non-expandable lung or trapped lung – with long-term dyspnoea due to progressive fibrosis. Rheumatoid nodules and interstitial lung disease are seen in up to 30%. Treatment usually involves NSAIDs initially followed by oral steroids (e.g. 10–20 mg prednisolone) tapered over a few weeks, whilst optimising maintenance RA therapy. For large/recurrent effusion-causing symptoms, thoracentesis ± IPC is a reasonable course of intervention. Benign asbestos-related pleural effusion, also known as BAPE, is included in the differential, but this should be a diagnosis of exclusion and would not typically cause chest pain.

The RA treatment was escalated to a combination of methotrexate, hydroxychloroquine and leflunomide. His IPC remained in place and continued to function well until approximately 18 months later when he attended a rheumatology outpatient follow-up appointment and mentioned that he was no longer getting as much benefit from the drainage and in addition to the breathlessness he was feeling 'giddy'. His legs felt weak and his ankles were swelling.

Thoracic ultrasound in the clinic showed gross visceral and parietal pleural thickening, parenchymal banding and a small amount of heavily septated fluid (Figure 4.3).

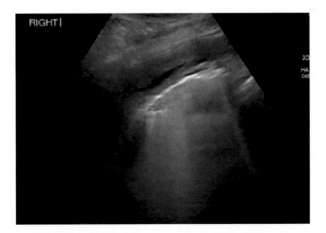

Figure 4.3 Right-sided thoracic ultrasound showing the presence of a small septated pleural effusion along with parietal and visceral pleural thickening.

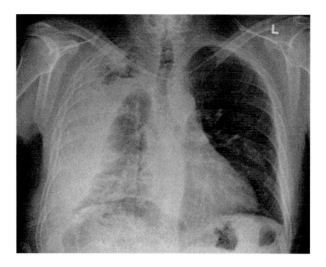

Figure 4.4 Chest radiograph showing the presence of a large, right-sided loculated effusion with the IPC in situ.

He was anaemic with an Hb 92 g/dL from a baseline of 105 g/dL, WCC 9,000/mm³ and CRP 17 mg/L, and BNP was elevated. Two weeks later, he presented with a cough, productive green phlegm, fevers and rigors, and was admitted. His WCC had gone up to 18,000/mm³ and his CRP was 222 mg/L. The pleural fluid from the IPC was sampled and was blood stained. Chest X-ray showed a large, right-sided loculated pleural effusion (Figure 4.4).

PF biochemistry – protein 42 g/dL, glucose <0.3 mmol/L, LDH 10,500 IU/L
PF microscopy and culture – methicillin-sensitive *Staphylococcus aureus* (from both standard culture bottles and BACTEC blood culture bottles)
PF cytology – acute inflammation, no evidence of malignancy

c) How do you define IPC-related infection and how does it differ from standard pleural infection?

The modified Delphi Consensus Statement (3) categorises IPC-related infectious complications into 'local' IPC-related infection defined as the presence of infectious signs/symptoms around the catheter site or tunnel tract such as tenderness or erythema. These may also include systemic signs of infection such as fever and leucocytosis.

The second category known as 'IPC-related pleural space infection' is defined as the presence of pus from the pleural space or the presence of gram stain or culture-positive pleural fluid with clinical signs of infection.

However, the diagnosis can be challenging. Low pH and high LDH in MPE with fevers due to underlying tumours are not uncommon. Bacterial colonisation of IPC can yield positive microbiology without clinical

manifestation of pleural infection, and studies are lacking regarding the significance of this in IPC-treated patients or the relevant bacteriology. A large
multicentre review of >1,000 patients from 11 centres found a true incidence
rate of infection of 4.8% (4). The most common organisms are *Staphylococcus
aureus*, *Pseudomonas aeruginosa* and Enterobacteria. Typical onset of infection is a minimum of 6–8 weeks after insertion, which goes against a direct
relation to the insertion procedure but rather highlights the importance of
catheter aftercare. The mortality of IPC-related pleural space infection is
generally low (0.3%) compared to community-acquired pleural infection.

The IPC was attached to an underwater seal with regular saline flushes. The
immunosuppressive medication for RA was withheld and oral clindamycin
and ciprofloxacin were commenced. Over the course of the following week, the
inflammatory markers settled and he was discharged home to complete a 6-week
course of antibiotics with a more frequent IPC drainage regimen and an interim
pleural clinic review 2 weeks after discharge.

Three months later, he presented acutely to the ED with breathlessness and
was hypoxic. Chest X-ray showed a large, right-sided hydropneumothorax with
dislodgement of the IPC (Figure 4.5). He had deteriorated from an exercise tolerance of 100 m on the flat to now getting breathless on transferring out of bed.

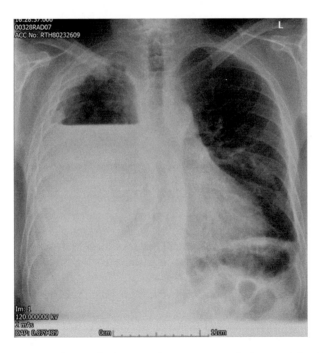

Figure 4.5 Chest radiograph showing the presence of a large, right-sided
hydropneumothorax.

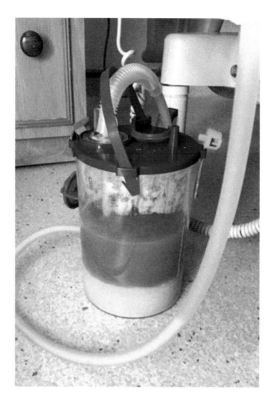

Figure 4.6 Chest tube drainage bottle showing the presence of pus.

The IPC had dislodged (presumed due to the pressure of the increasing amount of fluid). He was commenced on intravenous antibiotics and furosemide with a view to IPC re-insertion once stable.

Blood tests prior to the IPC procedure revealed Hb 68 g/dL, PT (Prothrombin time) 87 sec and INR 8.3. Further haematological testing and consultation suggested that he had an unexplained drop in factor VII levels presumably due to the underlying infection and inflammation. Discussion among the multidisciplinary team of the case in conjunction with the patient concluded that a drainage procedure was essential to control sepsis, and the patient consented to a high-risk IPC re-insertion (Figure 4.6). He received 2 units of RBCs (red blood cells) pre-procedure along with periprocedural IV tranexamic acid and underwent an uncomplicated IPC re-insertion and sampling of fluid.

PF biochemistry – protein 32 g/dL, glucose <0.3 mmol/L, LDH 22,300 IU/L
PF cytology – purulent brown fluid
PF micro – *Staphlococcus aureus* (resistant to ciprofloxacin)

He was discharged with a further 6-week course of clindamycin. On interim review 6 weeks later, he had improved with no fevers and was gaining weight. His exercise tolerance had improved back to 200–300 yards, haemoglobin was stable,

C-reactive protein (CRP) was downtrending and albumin was improving. There was little fluid now draining from the IPC. He remained off RA drugs and joint disease remained quiescent. Despite this, however, he had a low-grade tachycardia, ongoing right pleuritic chest pain, persistent septated effusion and what was now significant pleural fibrosis.

d) What are the further options for the management of this patient?

The treating team suspected that the IPC was blocked. Admission for fibrinolytics would normally be an appropriate course of action, but in this case, there was a particularly high risk for bleeding complications given the factor VII deficiency. This would likely require a modified reduced dosing regimen with careful observation if this were to be considered.

The other consideration was whether, in view of improving performance status, surgical options were now possible. A detailed discussion with thoracic surgery colleagues concluded that decortication via video-assisted thoracoscopic surgery (VATS) would have a very high risk of conversion to thoracotomy, and their preference was an open thoracotomy (Clagett procedure) with a residual open fistula to chronically drain the collection (Figure 4.7).

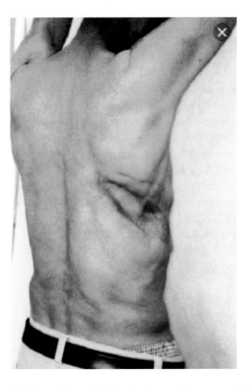

Figure 4.7 Clinical picture of a patient who has undergone a Clagett thoracotomy. An open window with resection of a posterolateral lower rib in the right posterolateral hemithorax is seen to allow drainage of the empyema.

Ultimately, the patient declined surgery and fibrinolytics were thought to be too high risk. There remained an underlying suspicion of the development of pleural malignancy. He, therefore, underwent a diagnostic and therapeutic medical thoracoscopy into a septated and fibrosed pleural space. A two-port technique was used to dissect and unify the pleural space. Pleural biopsies were undertaken and a new IPC was inserted. He was started on antibiotics and the decision was made for these to be continued long term in a 'month on–month off' cycle. His methotrexate was restarted. Four years later, he remains clinically well with a weekly drainage of 200 ml from his IPC and no chest pain. He is gardening, walking to shops regularly and planning a holiday.

## KEY POINTS

- In the context of RA, asbestos, cancer and heart failure, diagnosis of pleural infection is challenging.
- Pleural infection rarely presents as typical sepsis. Keep a high index of suspicion for 'slow burning' pleural infection with continually elevated inflammatory markers and features such as weight loss and reduced albumin reflecting a chronic catabolic state.
- IPC can be useful in achieving sepsis control in pleural infection, and prolonged courses of antibiotics are often required.
- Monitor these patients closely.

## REFERENCES

1. DePew ZS, Verma A, Wigle D, Mullon JJ, Nichols FC, Maldonado F. Nonspecific pleuritis: Optimal duration of follow-up. *Ann Thorac Surg* 2014;97(6):1867–1871.
2. Janssen J, Maldonado F, Metintas M. What is the significance of nonspecific pleuritis? A trick question. *Clin Respir J* 2018;12(9):2407–2410.
3. Gilbert CR, Wahidi MM, Light RW, et al. Management of indwelling tunneled pleural catheters: A modified Delphi consensus statement. *Chest* 2020;158(5):2221–2228.
4. Fysh ETH, Tremblay A, Feller-Kopman D, et al. Clinical outcomes of indwelling pleural catheter-related pleural infections: an international multicenter study. *Chest* 2013;144(5):1597–1602.

# 5

# To ambulate or admit?

EIHAB BEDAWI

A 68-year-old gentleman presented to the ambulatory assessment unit with a history of dry cough, left-sided chest discomfort and mild shortness of breath for approximately 3 weeks. He had received two courses of antibiotics in the community: first amoxicillin and then clarithromycin without clinical improvement. His wife was concerned, as he was also losing weight and off his food. He denied any fevers or night sweats and no haemoptysis.

His past history included non-insulin-dependent diabetes and atrial fibrillation for which he was on apixaban. He had a 20 pack-year smoking history but stopped 10 years prior to presentation. He was a retired civil servant with no significant occupational exposures and admitted to moderate EtOH excess.

Blood tests revealed a mildly raised WCC 13,100/mm$^3$, platelet 450,000/mm$^3$ and CRP 105 mg/L. His renal function demonstrated normal creatinine but a modestly raised urea of 9 mmol/L. His liver function was mildly deranged with an albumin of 28 g/L and modestly raised GGT. He underwent a chest radiograph, which is depicted in Figure 5.1.

His haemodynamic parameters were completely normal and the referring physician remarked that he looked clinically well. The referring team reported that he is keen to go home and they think he is suitable for ambulatory management. They, therefore, considered treating him with a broader spectrum oral agent (co-amoxiclav) and discharging him with a follow-up radiograph in 4 weeks.

A) Choose the correct option.
1) The most likely diagnosis is a left-sided, simple parapneumonic effusion. Given he is clinically stable, ambulating with oral co-amoxiclav is reasonable but he should have an earlier follow-up in 1–2 weeks.
2) The most likely diagnosis is a left-sided, complicated parapneumonic effusion. Given he is clinically stable, ambulating with oral co-amoxiclav is reasonable, but he should have an earlier follow-up in 1–2 weeks.

DOI: 10.1201/9781003081630-5

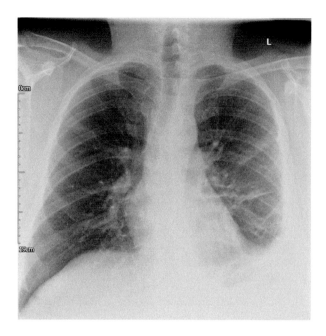

Figure 5.1 Chest X-ray showing the presence of a small, left-sided effusion.

3) The most likely diagnosis is a left-sided, complicated parapneumonic effusion. He requires urgent admission for intravenous antibiotics and urgent ultrasound-guided pleural tap ± chest tube insertion.

4) Given he is clinically stable, he can be discharged with oral antibiotics but should be given instructions to withhold his anticoagulation and return for an outpatient, ultrasound-guided pleural tap ± drain to exclude a complicated parapneumonic effusion.

This man has some worrying features in his presentation that are suggestive of a complicated parapneumonic effusion or pleural infection. His symptoms have been going on for 3 weeks, and he has failed two courses of antibiotics. Pleural infection does not always present with typical 'sepsis', and it is important to remember that the presentation, particularly in the older population, is often subacute with non-specific symptoms of general deterioration due to the ensuing catabolic state and the haemodynamic parameters can be normal. In this case, the symptom of left-chest discomfort provided an additional clue for underlying pleurisy.

A study by Chalmers et al. identified six clinical predictors of the development of a complicated parapneumonic effusion or pleural infection when presenting to hospital with a pneumonic presentation (Table 5.1). These included an albumin <30 g/L, CRP >100 mg/L, platelet count >400 × 10⁹/L, sodium <130 mmol/L, intravenous drug use and chronic alcohol abuse (1). This patient had four of these risk factors.

B) Assuming this gentleman has pleural infection, is there any way of predicting his prognosis as another method of risk stratification at the front door?

The RAPID score (Table 5.2) is prospectively derived and remains the only externally validated risk stratification tool specific to pleural infection (2, 3). It allows triage of patients with pleural infection to one of three categories – low, medium and high – with varying predicted mortalities at 3 months. Each of the RAPID tool variables is independently predictive, so in this patient, even without having seen, scanned or sampled the pleural collection, we have enough clinical information (based on serum urea, age,

Table 5.1 Clinical predictors of development of pleural infection

| Clinical feature | AOR (95% CI) | p Value |
|---|---|---|
| Albumin <30 g/L | 4.55 (2.45 to 8.45) | <0.0001 |
| CRP >100 mg/L | 15.7 (3.69 to 66.9) | 0.0002 |
| Platelet count >400 × 10$^9$/L | 4.09 (2.21 to 7.54) | <0.0001 |
| Sodium <130 mmol/L | 2.70 (1.55 to 4.70) | 0.0005 |
| Intravenous drug use | 2.82 (1.09 to 7.30) | 0.03 |
| Chronic alcohol abuse | 4.28 (1.87 to 9.82) | 0.0006 |

Source: Adapted from Table 4 in Chalmers JD, Singanayagam A, Murray MP, Scally C, Fawzi A, Hill AT, Risk factors for complicated parapneumonic effusion and empyema on presentation to hospital with community-acquired pneumonia, Thorax 2009 Jul;64(7):592–7.

Table 5.2 The RAPID scoring system

| Parameter | Measure | | Score |
|---|---|---|---|
| Renal | Urea | <5 mmol/L | 0 |
| | | 5–8 mmol/L | 1 |
| | | >8 mmol/L | 2 |
| Age | Age | <50 years | 0 |
| | | 50–70 years | 1 |
| | | >70 years | 2 |
| Purulence of fluid | Purulent | | 0 |
| | Non-purulent | | 1 |
| Infection source | Community acquired | | 0 |
| | Hospital acquired | | 1 |
| Dietary factors | Albumin | >27 mmol/L | 0 |
| | | <27 mmol/L | 1 |
| | | | |
| Risk categories | Score 0–2 | | Low risk |
| | Score 2–4 | | Medium risk |
| | Score 5–7 | | High risk |

infection source and serum albumin) to predict that his RAPID score is at least 4, putting him in the moderate category with a 3-month mortality of at least 10% and a 1-year mortality of 18% (Figure 5.2).

C) Are there any situations where pleural infection can be managed conservatively or using an ambulatory approach?

Small parapneumonic effusions that are <5 cm on an erect lateral chest X-ray (4) or <2.5 cm on CT scan (5) can be managed without thoracentesis, although where diagnostic sampling is feasible this may be helpful to confirm diagnosis and microbiology. A recent retrospective study confirmed that some patients with small pleural collections can be managed successfully with antibiotics alone with a slightly higher but statistically insignificant infection-related mortality rate (6). This suggests that for very small or difficult-to-access pleural infection collections, it may be possible in selected patients to treat with antibiotics alone without drainage of fluid, although early follow-up and regular review are recommended.

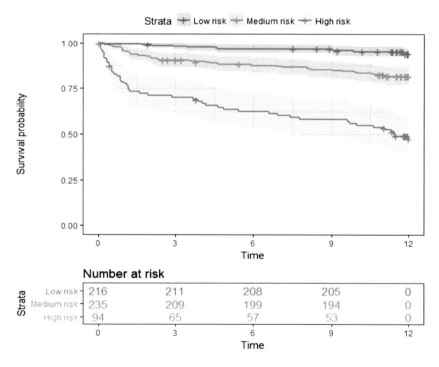

Figure 5.2 Kaplan–Meier graphs censored for loss to follow-up according to baseline RAPID risk category (based on a single representative imputed dataset). RAPID scores are 0–2 (low risk), 3–4 (medium risk) and 5–7 (high risk). Shaded areas represent 95% confidence intervals for survival at each point.

## PROGRESS

Based on the aforementioned evidence and clinical rationale, the team redis-cussed with the patient and he agreed to be admitted to the respiratory ward. He was commenced on intravenous antibiotics with co-amoxiclav and oral metro-nidazole to extend his anaerobic cover. He was started on intravenous fluids, and his apixaban was withheld and replaced with prophylactic low-molecular-weight heparin. He was prescribed nutritional supplements with a view to a formal dieti-tian review. He had an ultrasound scan conducted as follows (Figure 5.3).

A diagnostic tap was performed, demonstrating a pH of 6.9, glucose 0.1 mmol/L and LDH 3580 IU/L.

D) Based on the ultrasound appearance, what is the next best course of management?
   1) Small bore 12–14F chest tube
   2) Large bore (≥18F) chest tube
   3) Refer directly for medical thoracoscopy
   4) Refer directly for surgery

Radiological parameters predicting outcomes have been challenging to study in pleural infection, mostly because studies to date have been largely small, retrospective and have demonstrated that radiology tends to predict clinician behaviour rather than the true outcome from pleural infection (7–9).

The presence of sonographic septations, such as those in the ultrasound image in Figure 5.3, is often assumed to be associated with the need for more

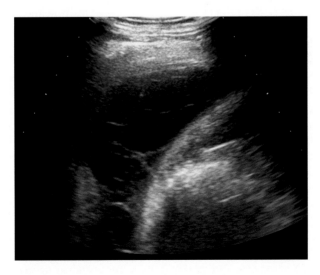

Figure 5.3 Thoracic ultrasound showing the presence of a moderate, left-sided pleural effusion with septations.

aggressive upfront drainage therapy such as intrapleural fibrinolytics or surgical drainage. However, the evidence linking this to worse outcomes in pleural infection is limited to small retrospective case series (8, 10). To date, the largest pleural infection trials (11, 12) were conducted prior to the era of commonplace ultrasound and hence the RAPID model did not address these. The only prospective study to specifically examine this did not find that sonographic septations were independently predictive of worse outcomes (13). Therefore, initial drainage with a chest tube should always be attempted.

Traditionally, large-bore chest drains have been used to drain pus or viscous fluid. A retrospective analysis of the MIST-1 RCT (n = 405) (12) is the only direct comparison study of chest tube size in pleural infection (14). Patients treated with a range of chest drain sizes (from <10 F to >20 F) showed no difference in primary and secondary outcomes (death, need for thoracic surgery, length of stay, chest radiograph appearance and lung function at 3 months) according to chest drain size. Moreover, large-bore chest drains were associated with more pain. These data, therefore, show that small-bore chest drains are sufficient as a first-line intervention for pleural infection. There is concern that smaller bore chest drains tend to become occluded with fibrin or pus. In the MIST-1 trial, chest tube patency was maintained with 3-times-daily 30 mL saline flushes. One retrospective study reported that only 1 out of 58 drains flushed with 20 mL sterile saline every 6 h became blocked (versus 6 out of 19 non-flushed drains) (15). Care is usually taken to ensure that all the fenestrations on the chest drain are located intrapleurally to work effectively and minimise the risk of infected fluid leakage into subcutaneous tissue.

Medical thoracoscopy is well established in the management of pleural effusion, however, its role in pleural infection is less clearly defined. Advocates of medical thoracoscopy have demonstrated success rates of 79.3%–97.7% in multi-loculated organising empyema (16–19). A recent meta-analysis of non-randomised studies reported a pooled treatment success rate of 85% when utilised as first-line therapy or after the failure of a chest tube, with a complication rate of 9% (20). Higher success rates were associated with bacteriological negative effusions and administration of adjuvant intrapleural fibrinolysis (20). A recent randomised controlled trial of medical thoracoscopy versus intrapleural fibrinolytic therapy showed a shorter length of stay post-intervention associated with the thoracoscopy arm (21). The small numbers within the trial and the limitations of the primary outcome require further studies to establish the true role of medical thoracoscopy in empyema.

The patient went on to have an optimally placed ultrasound-guided 12F chest tube placed under direct vision secured with an anchor stitch and a bespoke dressing followed by regular saline (30 ml tds) flushes. The patient made a good response to standard care and by day 3 had a tiny residual collection and the C-reactive protein (CRP) had dropped by more than 50% of the baseline value. The tube was removed on day 5, antibiotics were switched to oral and the patient was discharged on day 7 to complete a total of 4 weeks antibiotic therapy. He was reviewed in the outpatient clinic 2 weeks after discharge and again 2 months after discharge with complete resolution of symptoms and normalisation of chest X-ray/ultrasound appearances.

## KEY POINTS

- Prompt diagnosis and early treatment with pleural fluid drainage and antibiotic therapy are of paramount importance in improving patient outcomes with pleural infection.
- RAPID score can be used as a prognostic score to predict mortality at 3 months in patients with pleural infection.
- More research is needed to assess the role of upfront invasive procedures such as medical thoracoscopy and surgery.

## REFERENCES

1. Chalmers JD, Singanayagam A, Murray MP, Scally C, Fawzi A, Hill AT. Risk factors for complicated parapneumonic effusion and empyema on presentation to hospital with community-acquired pneumonia. *Thorax* 2009 July 1;64(7):592.
2. Rahman NM, Kahan BC, Miller RF, Gleeson FV, Nunn AJ, Maskell NA. A clinical score (RAPID) to identify those at risk for poor outcome at presentation in patients with pleural infection. *Chest* 2014 April;145(4):848–55.
3. Corcoran JP, Psallidas I, Gerry S, Piccolo F, Koegelenberg CF, Saba T, et al. Prospective validation of the RAPID clinical risk prediction score in adult patients with pleural infection: The PILOT study. *Eur Respir J* 2020 November;56(5):2000130.
4. Metersky ML. Is the lateral decubitus radiograph necessary for the management of a parapneumonic pleural effusion? *Chest* 2003 September;124(3):1129–32.
5. Moffett BK, Panchabhai TS, Anaya E, Nakamatsu R, Arnold FW, Peyrani P, et al. Computed tomography measurements of parapneumonic effusion indicative of thoracentesis. *Eur Respir J* 2011 December;38(6):1406–11.
6. Porcel JM, Valencia H, Bielsa S. Adult patients with parapneumonic empyema who may not require pleural drainage. *Rev Clin Esp (Barc)* 2016 April;216(3):172–4.
7. Kearney SE, Davies CW, Davies RJ, Gleeson FV. Computed tomography and ultrasound in parapneumonic effusions and empyema. *Clin Radiol* 2000 July;55(7):542–7.
8. Chen CH, Chen W, Chen HJ, Yu YH, Lin YC, Tu CY, et al. Transthoracic ultrasonography in predicting the outcome of small-bore catheter drainage in empyemas or complicated parapneumonic effusions. *Ultrasound Med Biol* 2009 September;35(9):1468–74.

9. Huang HC, Chang HY, Chen CW, Lee CH, Hsiue TR. Predicting factors for outcome of tube thoracostomy in complicated parapneumonic effusion for empyema. *Chest* 1999 March;115(3):751–6.

10. Chen HJ, Tu CY, Ling SJ, Chen W, Chiu KL, Hsia TC, et al. Sonographic appearances in transudative pleural effusions: Not always an anechoic pattern. *Ultrasound Med Biol* 2008 March;34(3):362–9.

11. Rahman NM, Maskell NA, West A, Teoh R, Arnold A, Mackinlay C, et al. Intrapleural use of tissue plasminogen activator and DNase in pleural infection. *N Engl J Med* 2011 August 11;365(6):518–26.

12. Maskell NA, Davies CWH, Nunn AJ, Hedley EL, Gleeson FV, Miller R, et al. U.K. controlled trial of intrapleural streptokinase for pleural infection. *N Engl J Med* 2005 March 3;352(9):865–74.

13. Bedawi EO, Kanellakis NI, Corcoran JP, Zhao Y, Hassan M, Asciak R, et al. The biological role of pleural fluid PAI-1 and sonographic septations in pleural infection: Analysis of a prospectively collected clinical outcome study. *Am J Respir Crit Care Med* 2022 October 3.

14. Rahman NM, Maskell NA, Davies CWH, Hedley EL, Nunn AJ, Gleeson FV, et al. The relationship between chest tube size and clinical outcome in pleural infection. *Chest* 2010 March;137(3):536–43.

15. Davies HE, Merchant S, McGown A. A study of the complications of small bore 'Seldinger' intercostal chest drains. *Respirology* 2008 June;13(4):603–7.

16. Ohuchi M, Inoue S, Ozaki Y, Fujita T, Igarashi T, Ueda K, et al. Single-trocar thoracoscopy under local anesthesia for pleural space infection. *Gen Thorac Cardiovasc Surg* 2014 August;62(8):503–10.

17. Hardavella G, Papakonstantinou NA, Karampinis I, Papavasileiou G, Ajab S, Shafaat M, et al. Hippocrates quoted 'if an empyema does not rupture, death will occur': Is medical thoracoscopy able to make it rupture safely? *J Bronchol Interv Pulmonol* 2017 January;24(1):15–20.

18. Tacconi F, Pompeo E, Fabbi E, Mineo TC. Awake video-assisted pleural decortication for empyema thoracis. *Eur J Cardio Thorac Surg* 2010 March;37(3):594–601.

19. Ravaglia C, Gurioli C, Tomassetti S, Casoni GL, Romagnoli M, Gurioli C, et al. Is medical thoracoscopy efficient in the management of multiloculated and organized thoracic empyema? *Respiration* 2012;84(3):219–24.

20. Mondoni M, Saderi L, Trogu F, Terraneo S, Carlucci P, Ghelma F, et al. Medical thoracoscopy treatment for pleural infections: A systematic review and meta-analysis. *BMC Pulm Med* 2021 April 20;21(1):127.

21. Kheir F, Thakore S, Mehta H, Jantz M, Parikh M, Chee A, et al. Intrapleural fibrinolytic therapy versus early medical thoracoscopy for treatment of pleural infection. Randomized controlled clinical trial. *Ann Am Thorac Soc* 2020 August;17(8):958–64.

# 6

# Right-sided pleural effusion in a young Nepalese man

RADHIKA BANKA

A 22-year-old Nepalese man presented to the pleural service with a 6-week history of evening temperatures, right-sided pleuritic chest pain, dry cough, weight loss of 4 kilograms and loss of appetite. His brother with whom he shared the household was diagnosed with pulmonary multidrug-resistant tuberculosis (TB) 6 months prior and was on second-line anti-tuberculous treatment.

He was initially evaluated at another hospital 2 weeks after symptom onset. A chest radiograph demonstrated a right pleural effusion. He underwent diagnostic and therapeutic ultrasound-guided pleural aspiration where 800 ml of straw-coloured fluid was aspirated. The pleural fluid characteristics were protein 4.5 g/dL, LDH 800 IU/L, 75% lymphocytic and glucose 0.8 mmol/L. This was suggestive of an exudative pleural effusion. A pleural fluid aerobic culture did not demonstrate growth and the pleural fluid TB PCR (polymerase chain reaction) was negative. The pleural fluid TB culture was negative.

a) What is the pathophysiology of a tuberculous pleural effusion?

Tuberculous pleural effusion (TPE) is the second most common form of extrapulmonary tuberculosis (after lymphatic invasion) and is the most common cause of pleural effusion in TB-endemic countries. TPE usually occurs due to the rupture of a subpleural parenchymal focus into the pleural space. This causes an inflammatory reaction leading to increased pleural fluid formation. The initial inflammatory response is neutrophilic, which is then followed by lymphocytic inflammation, which leads to the release of adenosine deaminase and formation of granulomas. Granulomatous involvement of the pleura leads to obstruction of the pleural lymphatics and hence pleural fluid clearance is impaired.

DOI: 10.1201/9781003081630-6

TPE was initially thought to be a delayed hypersensitivity reaction to the tuberculin antigen, however, it is now possible to culture *Mycobacterium tuberculosis* (MTB) from either pleural fluid or pleural tissue in 70% cases and hence is now presumed to be a paucibacillary tuberculous infection within the pleural space (1).

b) What pleural fluid biomarkers aid in diagnosing tuberculous pleural effusion?

TPE is usually an exudative effusion with raised protein and lactate dehydrogenase (LDH) with characteristically low glucose levels. Differential cell count reveals a lymphocytic effusion (>50%), with less than 5% mesothelial cells. Neutrophils may predominate in the first few days of the effusion. Adenosine deaminase (ADA) is an important pleural biomarker for TPE diagnosis. ADA is a purine-degrading enzyme predominantly found in lymphocytes. It has two isoforms: ADA1, which is found in all cells but particularly in lymphocytes and monocytes; and ADA2, which is found only in monocytes. ADA2 is the predominant isoform in TPE. The primary utility of ADA lies in the detection of TPE in low-prevalence settings for its negative predictive value. The optimum cut-off used for ADA for diagnosing TPE has been much debated. A recent meta-analysis has shown that at a cut-off of 40 U/L, ADA has a sensitivity of 0.92 and a specificity of 0.9 with a negative predictive value of 0.93 (range: 0.98 at a 20% prevalence to 0.93 at a 60% prevalence setting) for diagnosing TPE. In general, pleural fluid ADA levels greater than 70 U/L are highly suggestive of TPE, and ADA levels below 40 U/L are helpful in excluding TPE. ADA may also be raised in other effusions due to other conditions such as rheumatoid arthritis, bacterial infections, lung cancer and haematological malignancies especially lymphoma (2).

He was presumptively diagnosed with TPE and commenced on an empiric weight-adjusted anti-tuberculous treatment with rifampicin, isoniazid, pyrazinamide and ethambutol. However, treatment did not result in symptom reduction after 1 month. A repeat chest radiograph demonstrated worsening of the right pleural effusion and he was referred to the pleural service. Ultrasound showed the presence of a heterogeneously septated, echoic pleural effusion with smooth parietal pleural thickening spanning over three rib spaces (Figure 6.1).

c) What is the role of radiology in diagnosing tuberculous pleural effusion?

Chest radiographs usually demonstrate the presence of a unilateral small to moderate pleural effusion. Computed tomography (CT) may demonstrate parenchymal lesions in the form of cavitation or subpleural nodules in addition to the presence of an effusion; various studies have shown parenchymal involvement ranging from 40% to 80%. CT can also be used to assess TB empyema where it shows thickened parietal and visceral pleura separated by fluid, known as the split pleura sign. Ultrasound findings in TPE range from anechoic to homogeneously echoic to a complex septated effusion. There is some evidence to suggest that loculations in the effusion are associated with culture positivity for MTB. Ultrasound is useful for the detection of pleural thickening and other pleural abnormalities, which can aid the operator find a preferred biopsy site.

He underwent ultrasound-guided pleural biopsies with an 18G cutting needle with pleural fluid aspiration. Histopathology showed the presence of caseating granulomas (Figure 6.2), and TB PCR from the pleural biopsies confirmed the presence of MTB with rifampicin resistance, indicating the presence of

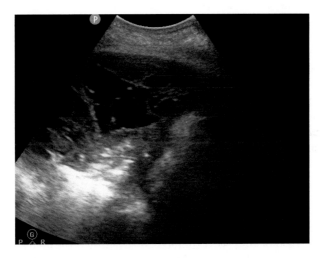

Figure 6.1  Right ultrasound image showing a septated pleural effusion.

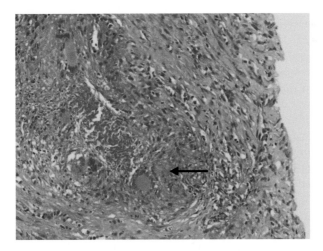

Figure 6.2  Haematoxylin and eosin stain of the parietal pleura showing the presence of necrotising granulomatous inflammation (black arrow).

multidrug-resistant tuberculosis. He was commenced on second-line anti-tuberculous treatment, which was then modified according to the drug susceptibility pattern obtained from the positive pleural tissue TB culture.

d) What is the role of ultrasound-guided and thoracoscopic biopsies for TPE diagnosis?

Microbiological confirmation of TPE with either microscopy, TB culture or TB PCR tests is of paramount importance with the increasing prevalence of drug-resistant TB. Unfortunately, the microbiological yield of pleural fluid for TPE remains poor. The sensitivity of TB microscopy, liquid TB culture and TB PCR tests for pleural fluid is 10%, 30%–60% and 40%–58%, respectively (3). Hence, in those with a high clinical suspicion of TB, a pleural biopsy with culture needs to be pursued to achieve a definitive diagnosis. Pleural biopsies can be obtained by either closed biopsies (with or without ultrasound guidance) or pleuroscopy. The diagnostic yield of blind pleural biopsies using Abram's needle has ranged from 48% to 93% for microbiological diagnosis of TPE. Given its simplicity and cost-effectiveness, it is still an attractive option in TB-endemic low-resource settings. The current British Thoracic Society (BTS) guidelines advise against blind pleural biopsy in low TPE prevalence settings with low operator experience. Ultrasound-guided pleural biopsies have gained more popularity in the past few years, with the advantage of direct ultrasound vision as compared to blind pleural biopsies. Given the diffuse involvement of the parietal pleura due to TB, ultrasound-guided pleural biopsies have a high diagnostic yield of 90% (4). A thoracoscopic biopsy is the gold standard for diagnosis of TPE and various studies have shown diagnostic yield at nearly 100%. It also provides the additional advantage of breaking septations and completely draining the fluid. The endoscopic picture at thoracoscopy shows the presence of diffuse small parietal nodularity, hyperaemia, septations and thickening of the parietal pleura. It is a safe procedure which can be performed on an outpatient basis, however, is limited by its availability in low-resource settings.

e) What is the treatment for tuberculous pleural effusion?

Treatment of TPE primarily involves anti-tuberculous therapy. Standard, drug-sensitive TPE is treated for 6 months, comprised of an intensive phase with a four-drug regime of rifampicin, isoniazid, pyrazinamide and ethambutol for 2 months followed by a continuation phase comprised of rifampicin and isoniazid for 4 months. Drug-resistant TPE is treated with second-line drugs based on drug susceptibility patterns, and treatment is usually recommended for 18–24 months. There is no role for routine use of corticosteroids in the management of TPE. Since most patients respond well to anti-tubercular treatment, the surgical role in TPE management is limited. It is reserved in TB empyema or residual pleural thickening that persists post-treatment leading to a fibrothorax and functional limitation (5).

## KEY POINTS

- The diagnosis of TPE should be suspected in patients with pleural effusion and relevant epidemiologic risk factors (previous history of TB infection, immunosuppression, diabetes mellitus, residence in or travel to a TB-endemic area).
- Diagnosis of TPE may be definitively established via demonstration of MTB in pleural fluid or a pleural biopsy specimen. Attempts should be made at obtaining pleural tissue for TPE diagnosis, as it increases diagnostic yield. This can be obtained by either ultrasound-guided or thoracoscopic pleural biopsies. Biopsies should be sent for histopathology, TB culture and TB PCR.
- TPE treatment mainly involves anti-tuberculous therapy. There is some evidence to suggest early and therapeutic pleural drainage may result in lesser residual pleural thickening and preserved lung function, however, more data is needed to establish this.

## REFERENCES

1. Seibert AF, Haynes J Jr, Middleton R, et al. Tuberculous pleural effusion. Twenty-year experience. *Chest* 1991;99(4):883–886.
2. Aggarwal AN, Agarwal R, Sehgal IS, Dhooria S. Adenosine deaminase for diagnosis of tuberculous pleural effusion: A systematic review and meta-analysis. *PLOS ONE* 2019 March 26;14(3):e0213728.
3. Kohli M, Schiller I, Dendukuri N, Yao M, Dheda K, Denkinger CM, Schumacher SG, Steingart KR. Xpert MTB/RIF Ultra and Xpert MTB/RIF assays for extrapulmonary tuberculosis and rifampicin resistance in adults. *Cochrane Database of Systematic Reviews* 2021(1): CD012768.
4. Koegelenberg CF, Irusen EM, von Groote-Bidlingmaier F et al. The utility of ultrasound-guided thoracentesis and pleural biopsy in undiagnosed pleural exudates. *Thorax* 2015;70(10):995–997.
5. Vorster MJ, Allwood BW, Diacon AH, Koegelenberg CF. Tuberculous pleural effusions: Advances and controversies. *J Thorac Dis* 2015;7(6):981–991.

# 7

# Bilateral transudative effusions

POPPY DENNISTON

An 80-year-old woman was referred to the pleural service with progressive breathlessness. She had a background of hypertrophic cardiomyopathy, atrial fibrillation with previous coronary artery bypass grafting, and chronic kidney disease (stage 3). Her medication included ramipril 5 mg twice daily, furosemide 80 mg in the morning and 40 mg at lunch, warfarin, and a LABA/ICS inhaler. She was an ex-smoker with a 10 pack-year history and a retired radiographer.

She had a chest X-ray (Figure 7.1) and subsequent CT chest which showed bilateral effusions, right more than left. On the thoracic CT scan, there was ground glass in the right-upper lobe and low-volume normal-shaped mediastinal lymphadenopathy.

a) How should we initially manage her right-sided effusion?

Pleural effusion in heart failure is very common; a prospective study found 87% of patients with decompensated heart failure requiring diuretics had pleural effusion (1). These may be unilateral or bilateral, and although slightly more common on the right, the presence of a left-sided unilateral effusion in a clinical context suggestive of cardiac failure does not necessarily warrant more invasive investigation (2). Initial treatment of heart failure–associated effusions is medical, often including ACE inhibitors, diuretics and beta blockers. The majority (>80%) of these effusions will respond to initial diuretic therapy and do not require drainage (1).

This patient is already under a cardiologist and is on appropriate medication, but despite this, the pleural fluid persists. A diagnostic and therapeutic aspiration is therefore warranted to confirm the suspected diagnosis, assess symptom relief following aspiration and ascertain if there is evidence of non-expansile lung which will guide future interventions.

 DOI: 10.1201/9781003081630-7

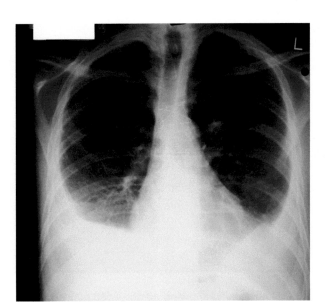

Figure 7.1 Chest radiograph showing bilateral effusion.

Given her breathlessness and asymmetrical moderate effusion, a diagnostic and therapeutic aspiration was performed (Figure 7.2). Approximately 700 mL of straw-coloured fluid was aspirated from the right side with the following investigation parameters:

| | |
|---|---|
| Protein | 24 g/dl |
| Glucose | 6 mmol/L |
| LDH | 74 IU/L |
| Cytology | Benign mesothelial cells and chronic inflammatory cells |
| Acid-fast bacillus/microbiology | No cells or organisms seen; no growth of acid-fast bacilli or microorganisms after culture |

Following the initial aspiration, the diuretic dose was increased. However, on review 2 weeks later, she reported ongoing breathlessness and was reviewed again by the pleural service. A repeat ultrasound scan showed a small, one-rib-space, 6 cm effusion and was not thought to be significantly contributing to her symptoms, thus further aspiration was not conducted, with dyspnoea assigned to likely cardiac function rather than pleural disease.

Six months later, she was re-referred with a larger effusion and was symptomatic with breathlessness. Ultrasound demonstrated a large right-sided pleural effusion, and she was scheduled for further aspiration. A further 700 mL of

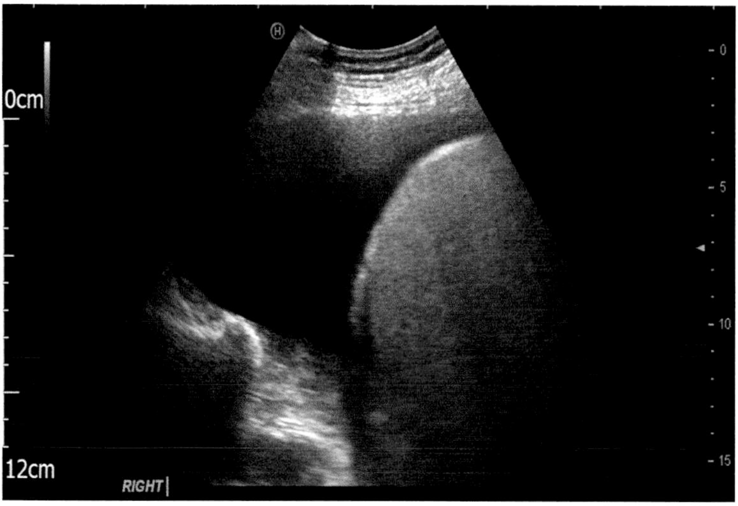

Figure 7.2 Thoracic ultrasound showing a right-sided non-echogenic pleural effusion.

straw-coloured fluid was aspirated, again demonstrating transudative biochemistry and bland cytology.

b) How should the transudative effusion now be managed?

Treatment of the underlying cause should be optimised, be that heart, kidney or renal failure, or other rarer causes. However, a detailed discussion of this is outside the remit of this case. Interventional management of refractory, non-malignant, transudative effusions focuses on symptom relief, as the accumulation of pleural fluid may have a significant effect on functional state of comorbid patients such as seen here. Similar strategies may be adopted to those in malignant pleural effusion, although there is a paucity of high-quality data.

Repeated therapeutic thoracentesis is a reasonable initial approach, but acceptability to the patient and clinician may depend on the rapidity of re-accumulation of fluid and the level of symptoms between drainages. Each procedure comes with the risk of infection or bleeding, and may require temporary cessation of anticoagulants or antiplatelets. It is postulated that the presence of pleural fluid may result in pleural thickening and therefore increase the risk of lung entrapment and resultant symptoms (3), although there exist no large studies confirming this.

Following the second aspiration, she reported improvement in breathing, but this lasted for only a few days before effusion and symptom recurrence. Further management options were discussed, and the patient opted for admission for a chest drain and talc slurry pleurodesis.

c) What is the role of talc pleurodesis in transudative effusions?

Large multicentre trials have established talc pleurodesis (whether slurry or poudrage) as an effective and safe management option for malignant pleural effusion. Its role in non-malignant disease is less certain. A large, single-centre retrospective study reported successful pleurodesis rates of 77% with talc poudrage (47/68 patients), however, the causes of the effusions were not established (4). These rates are replicated in other retrospective cohort studies where pleurodesis rates of 75%–80% (5,6) are reported.

Two weeks after intervention, the talc slurry pleurodesis was unsuccessful, with re-accumulation of fluid. She was noted to be increasingly frail and found travel to hospital for procedures tiring.

d) How should we proceed next? Is there a role for an indwelling pleural catheter (IPC)?

Treatment to date has been based on palliation and relief of symptoms, including the use of methods proven to be effective in malignant pleural effusion. IPCs have been shown to be an effective and safe option in malignant effusion, although the supportive data in non-malignant effusions is less clear (7,8). This evidence has generally been based on retrospective cohort reviews assessing outcomes and complications of IPCs. One large study found similar rates of complication and auto-pleurodesis as in a malignant pleural effusion group (7).

The best evidence comes from the recent REDUCE study, which was a multicentre, randomised controlled trial (RCT) investigating the effect on breathlessness of IPCs versus therapeutic thoracentesis (TT) over 12 weeks in non-malignant pleural effusion, specifically focusing on transudative effusions caused by cardiac, renal or hepatic failure. No significant difference in breathlessness was found between the two groups, despite the IPC group draining approximately 17 litres in their remaining life, and TT patients requiring only about three procedures. Significant complications were noted with IPCs including hypoalbuminaemia and an increased risk of infection (9). A follow-up RCT by the same group is currently underway assessing the role of therapeutic thoracentesis versus IPC and talc pleurodesis, specifically in heart failure, which may shed more light on the efficacy and safety of pleural interventions in the management of transudative effusions.

Based on this evidence, in our practice we tend to use IPCs only in patients who have demonstrated the need for regular repeat thoracentesis (usually more than three) or in whom repeat thoracentesis is difficult (due to required anticoagulation, complications or travel issues as here).

It is important to highlight the role of the multidisciplinary team in complex, deteriorating patients. In patients with significant symptoms and frailty, involvement of the community palliative care team, alongside specialist input for their primary organ failure, is necessary to provide holistic and comprehensive treatment for their symptoms.

The patient opted for an IPC. This was drained by the district nurses approximately 350 mL twice a week with good symptomatic relief. She was referred to local palliative care teams, as she had deteriorated significantly and required extra support and symptom control at home.

## KEY POINTS

- Transudative effusions from heart failure can be bilateral but may present as unilateral effusions.
- Optimisation of the underlying disease (cardiac failure or other) is key to optimal management.
- Once optimised, if pleural effusions persist and are symptomatic, repeat thoracentesis is an option to be considered. Talc pleurodesis often fails, but IPCs should only be used in selected patients after discussion about the relative risks and benefits.

## REFERENCES

1. Kataoka H. Pericardial and Pleural Effusions in Decompensated Chronic Heart Failure. *Am Heart J.* 2000;139(5):918–923.
2. Woodring JH. Distribution of pleural effusion in congestive heart failure: what is atypical?. *South Med J.* 2005;98(5): 518–523
3. Bintcliffe OJ, Lee GYC, Rahman NM, Maskell NA. The Management of Benign Non-infective Pleural Effusions. *Eur Respir Rev.* 2016;25(141):303–316.
4. Steger V, Mika U, Toomes H, et al. Who Gains Most? A 10-Year Experience With 611 Thoracoscopic Talc Pleurodeses. *Ann Thorac Surg.* 2007;83(6):1940–1945.
5. Glazer M, Berkman N, Lafair JS, Kramer MR. Successful Talc Slurry Pleurodesis in Patients with Nonmalignant Pleural Effusion. *Chest.* 2000;117(5):1404–1409.
6. Sudduth CD, Sahn SA. Pleurodesis for Nonmalignant Pleural Effusions: Recommendations. *Chest.* 1992;102(6):1855–1860.
7. Mullon J, Maldonado F. Use of Tunneled Indwelling Pleural Catheters for Palliation of Nonmalignant Pleural Effusions. *Chest.* 2011;140(4):996A.
8. Patil M, Dhillon SS, Attwood K, Saoud M, Alraiyes AH, Harris K. Management of Benign Pleural Effusions Using Indwelling Pleural Catheters: A Systematic Review and Meta-analysis. *Chest.* 2017;151(3):626–635.

9. Walker SP, Bintcliffe O, Keenan E, et al. Randomised Trial of Indwelling Pleural Catheters for Refractory Transudative Pleural Effusions. *Eur Respir J.* 2022;59(2):2101362.

# 8

# Renal failure and pleural fluid

ANAND SUNDARALINGAM

A 70-year-old woman with end-stage kidney disease (ESKD) was referred by the nephrologists to the interventional pulmonology (IP) service with cough and dyspnoea. The initial chest X-ray is shown in Figure 8.1.

a) What are the causes of pleural effusion in patients with ESKD?

Patients with ESKD may develop pleural effusions for many reasons. The estimated prevalence of pleural effusions in patients with ESKD is 22.6% (95% CI 21.3%–24%) [1–11].

These may relate to imbalances in hydrostatic and oncotic pressures, as a result of cardiac failure, hypervolaemia, or hypoalbuminaemia, or may be secondary to pleural inflammation as a result of uraemia or an underlying autoimmune aetiology that precipitated ESKD. Such patients are also at risk of pleural infection or malignancy, particularly if receiving immunosuppression, as might be the case in a post-renal transplant population. More unusual causes are also recognised, often relating to anatomical abnormalities or mechanical disruptions, such as pleuroperitoneal leakage through diaphragmatic porosities, or arteriovenous graft stenoses.

The patient had a diagnosis of Goodpasture's disease with a rapidly progressive nephropathy that had led to her becoming dialysis dependent. She had been managed for 12 months with haemodialysis but had decided to transition to peritoneal dialysis (PD) a month prior to her presentation to the IP service. Other medical history included mitral regurgitation following a myocardial infarction, hypertension and a mild COVID-19 infection 6 months prior to presentation. On clinical examination, she appeared euvolaemic.

DOI: 10.1201/9781003081630-8

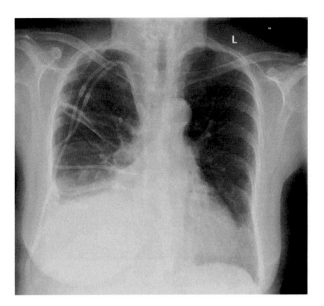

Figure 8.1  Initial chest X-ray with right-sided pleural effusion.

A diagnostic pleural aspiration was performed:

| | |
|---|---|
| Pleural fluid protein | <8 g/L |
| Serum protein | 67 g/L |
| Pleural fluid lactate dehydrogenase | <30 IU/L |
| Serum lactate dehydrogenase | 249 IU/L |
| Pleural fluid glucose | 5.5 mmol/L |
| Serum glucose | 4.9 mmol/L |

b) What does the pleural fluid biochemistry show and how would you interpret these findings, given the clinical context?

The pleural fluid biochemistry demonstrates a transudative effusion. Using Light's criteria, the ratio of pleural fluid (PF) protein to serum protein is <0.5 and the ratio of PF lactate dehydrogenase (LDH) to serum LDH is <0.6 and less than two-thirds of the upper limit of normal. What's more, the PF biochemistry shows features of an 'extreme' transudate, suggesting the pathophysiology was very unlikely to be secondary to pleural inflammation and more in keeping with an ultrafiltrate. Of note, the PF glucose exceeded that of serum.

Differential diagnoses could therefore include hypervolaemia, cardiac failure, hypoalbuminaemia or a pleuroperitoneal leak. Whilst she is at risk

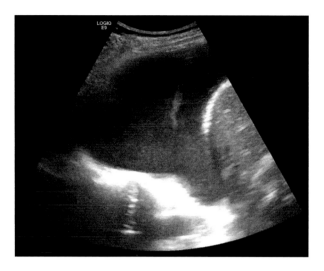

Figure 8.2 Thoracic ultrasound image showing recurrence of effusion.

for all of these conditions, the clinical presentation of euvolaemia and unilateral effusion, and the finding of an ultrafiltrate and PF glucose exceeding that of serum suggested this may be a pleuroperitoneal leak.

PD-associated pleuroperitoneal leak is a rare complication of peritoneal dialysis. In a large series by Nomoto et al., it was observed in 1.6% of all PD patients [12]. It describes the phenomenon of dialysate fluid translocating from the peritoneum into the pleural space via diaphragmatic defects.

In a study by Chow et al., they found that a PF glucose > serum glucose by 2.8 mmol/L had 100% specificity for diagnosing a pleuroperitoneal leak [13].

The patient was advised to suspend their PD and switch back to haemodialysis for a period of 6 weeks. Following this break, PD was cautiously re-introduced, and the patient was regularly monitored by the IP team. Two weeks after commencing PD, a thoracic ultrasound demonstrated a recurrence of effusion (Figure 8.2).

c) What are the options for monitoring a patient with a suspected PD-associated pleuroperitoneal leak?

Whilst thoracic ultrasound will be the most helpful tool in monitoring for the recurrence of PD-associated leak, one can use other measurements, particularly if the patient is being remotely followed-up. The patient may of course report dyspnoea, but this is a late sign and indicates a significant volume of fluid build-up. Other helpful measurements include a daily weight chart as the patient recommences PD, as well as monitoring the input/output of the PD catheter, expecting a neutral balance. These may be more sensitive, early indicators of a recurrent leak and should warrant further assessment with thoracic ultrasound.

d) What are the management options for PD-associated pleuroperitoneal leaks?

There is sparse evidence to guide optimal management of this unusual condition. It is prudent to be confident you are indeed managing a PD-associated leak. As described earlier, patients with ESKD remain at risk for pleural infection or malignancy, even in the absence of immunosuppressive agents, as ESKD itself is a form of immunoparesis.

If the pleural fluid biochemistry is not entirely diagnostic for a leak, additional investigations using tracer agents such as D-lactate, methylene blue, indigo, Omnipaque or 99Tc-labelled albumin can be used in the dialysate and are detectable in the PF through biochemical analysis or radiological imaging. However, these additional investigative steps are often not required, as the clinician can simply map the behaviour of the effusion through cessation and resumption of the PD.

The rationale for resting the patient from PD for a period of 6 weeks is to allow any diaphragmatic defects to heal. Across a number of case series, 53% did not recur after such a rest period and recommencing PD [14–16]. If recurrence is encountered following the resumption of PD, the clinician and patient are now faced with several options. All decisions must include the treating nephrologist and patient. If haemodialysis or renal transplant are considered preferable alternative interventions to definitive effusion control, then these should be offered instead.

If, however, PD is the preferred modality for renal replacement, then clinicians have the usual options available to them for definitive effusion control: indwelling pleural catheters (IPCs), chemical pleurodesis via intercostal drain and slurry or thoracoscopy and poudrage, or mechanical pleurodesis via thoracic surgery and repair of diaphragmatic defects.

Given the likelihood of persistent high-volume drain output and the risk of complications such as infection, the authors would not advocate an IPC in this population.

It is worth noting that patients with PD-associated pleuroperitoneal leak have normal, healthy pleura and, therefore, bedside pleurodesis attempts will result in significantly more discomfort than in those with diseased pleura (i.e. as found in malignant pleural disease). Therefore, one should pay particular attention to analgesia requirements if pursuing this approach.

The patient preferred to remain on PD as opposed to haemodialysis and, therefore, elected for a chest drain and talc slurry; this was arranged. The procedure was complicated by severe chest pain and discomfort, which required escalated doses of analgesia and input from the anaesthetic team. The patient was discharged and reviewed as an outpatient 6 weeks after discharge. Thoracic ultrasound during this encounter suggested sluggish lung sliding, consistent with partial pleurodesis. Therefore, PD was cautiously re-introduced, but unfortunately, the patient began noticing a diminished PD catheter output and a recurrence of her dyspnoea. Reassessment with a thoracic ultrasound confirmed a recurrence of effusion and therefore pleurodesis failure.

e) How would you now manage this patient?

Video-assisted thoracoscopic surgery (VATS) is superior at preventing recurrence when compared to chest drain and talc slurry in this population (88% resolution vs 48%), and therefore in suitable patients should be offered first-line [16]. However, given the patient's comorbidities, this wasn't initially pursued and, given the prior attempts at pleurodesis, may now be more challenging to undertake.

In collaboration with the nephrologists, it was decided to continue with haemodialysis and avoid further pleural interventions. The patient has since been assessed for a renal transplant and is on the waiting list for surgery.

## KEY POINTS

- There are several different causes for pleural effusion in the ESKD population and these should all be given due consideration before settling on PD-associated pleuroperitoneal leak as the underlying cause.
- Pleural fluid biochemistry will often be highly suggestive of a PD-associated leak. Although further confirmatory tests are available, they are rarely required.
- Observing the behaviour of the pleural effusion in response to stopping and starting PD may be the most effective tool in diagnosis.
- Identify early into the disease course, in collaboration with the nephrologists and the patient, which treatment modalities, from both a pleural and renal perspective, are suitable before settling on a management plan.
- A more invasive surgical intervention, up front, may be more suitable in some individuals given the greater success rate at reducing recurrence and the ability to better optimise analgesia requirements.

## REFERENCES

1. Lakadamyali H, Lakadamyali H, Ergun T. Thorax CT findings in symptomatic hemodialysis patients. *Transplant Proc.* 2008;40(1):71–76.
2. Jarratt MJ, Sahn SA. Pleural effusions in hospitalized patients receiving long-term hemodialysis. *Chest.* 1995;108(2):470–474.
3. Bakirci T, Sasak G, Ozturk S, Akcay S, Sezer S, Haberal M. Pleural effusion in long-term hemodialysis patients. *Transplant Proc.* 2007;39(4):889–891.
4. Coşkun M, Boyvat F, Bozkurt B, Agildere AM, Niron EA. Thoracic CT findings in long-term hemodialysis patients. *Acta Radiol Stockh Swed.* 1999;40(2) 1987:181–186.
5. Qureshi SQ, Idrees MK, Ahmad S, Ahmed E. Pleural effusion among patients on maintenance hemodialysis at SIUT Karachi, Pakistan. *Rawal Med J.* 2016;41:11–11.

6. Hamada S, Sano T, Nagatani Y, Tsukino M. Pleural effusion negatively impacts survival of patients undergoing maintenance hemodialysis. *Pulmonology*. 2019;25(1):58–60.
7. Shaik L, Thotamgari SR, Kowtha P, Ranjha S, Shah RN, Kaur P, Subramani R, Katta RR Mukhtadir Kalaiger A, Singh R A spectrum of pulmonary complications occurring in end-stage renal disease patients on maintenance hemodialysis. *Cureus* 13(6):e15426.
8. Jabbar A, Qureshi R, Nasir K, Dhrolia M, Ahmad A. Transudative and exudative pleural effusion in chronic kidney disease patients: A prospective single-center study. *Cureus*. 2021;13(10):e18649.
9. Ray S, Mukherjee S, Ganguly J, Abhishek K, Mitras S, Kundu S. A cross-sectional prospective study of pleural effusion among cases of chronic kidney disease. *Indian J Chest Dis Allied Sci*. 2013;55(4):209–213.
10. Uzan G, İkitimur H. Pleural effusion in end stage renal failure patients. *Sisli Etfal Hastan Tip Bul*. 2019;53(1):54–57.
11. Pant P, Baniya S, Jha A. Prevalence of respiratory manifestations in chronic kidney diseases; A descriptive cross-sectional study in A tertiary care hospital of Nepal. *JNMA J Nepal Med Assoc*. 2019;57(216):80–83.
12. Nomoto Y, Suga T, Nakajima K, Sakai H, Osawa G, Ota K, Kawaguchi Y, Sakai T, Sakai S, Shibata M. Acute hydrothorax in continuous ambulatory peritoneal dialysis--A collaborative study of 161 centers. *Am J Nephrol*. 1989;9(5):363–367.
13. Chow KM, Szeto CC, Wong TY-H, Li PK-T. Hydrothorax complicating peritoneal dialysis: Diagnostic value of glucose concentration in pleural fluid aspirate. *Perit Dial Int J Int Soc Perit Dial*. 2002;22(4):525–528.
14. Allen SM, Matthews HR. Surgical treatment of massive hydrothorax complicating continuous ambulatory peritoneal dialysis. *Clin Nephrol*. 1991;36(6):299–301.
15. Ramon RG, Carrasco AM. Hydrothorax in peritoneal dialysis. *Perit Dial Int*. 1998;18(1):5–10.
16. Chow KM, Szeto CC, Li PK-T. Management options for hydrothorax complicating peritoneal dialysis. *Semin Dial*. 2003;16(5):389–394.

# 9

# Management of pleural effusion in a patient with known liver disease

MOHAMED ELLAYEH

A 52-year-old female presented to the respiratory department with complaints of progressive shortness of breath over 3 weeks associated with alcohol-related liver cirrhosis, oesophageal varices, portal hypertension and a history of type 2 diabetes mellitus. On examination, the patient was distressed, jaundiced and had a distended abdomen. Auscultation revealed decreased breath sound on the right side. Chest X-ray showed a large, right-sided pleural effusion (Figure 9.1). Thoracic ultrasound showed the presence of a large, anechoic, non-septated, right-sided pleural effusion (Figure 9.2). She underwent a diagnostic and therapeutic pleural aspiration where 1.5 litres of pleural fluid was aspirated. Pleural aspiration demonstrated a transudate with low protein and lactate dehydrogenase (LDH), normal glucose and cytology/microbiology negative. Given the clinical presentation and pleural fluid analysis, a diagnosis of hepatic hydrothorax was made.

a. What is the mechanism of development of hepatic hydrothorax?

Hepatic hydrothorax (HH) is defined as the presence of an effusion with underlying chronic liver disease, without evidence of other cardiopulmonary disorders. It can be seen in 5%–15% of patients with advanced liver disease and is associated with significant morbidity and mortality (1). In the absence of a liver transplant, hepatic hydrothorax is associated with a median survival of 1 year from diagnosis (2).

Ascites secondary to liver cirrhosis occur due to portal hypertension, vasodilatation of splanchnic and systemic arteries, and activation of various neurohormonal pathways leading to decreased sodium and water excretion.

DOI: 10.1201/9781003081630-9

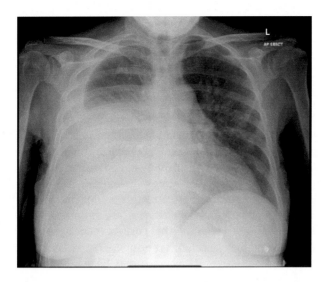

Figure 9.1  Initial chest X-ray showing a large, right-sided pleural effusion.

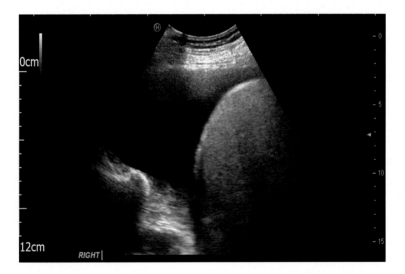

Figure 9.2  Ultrasound image showing a right-sided pleural effusion.

This leads to increased intra-abdominal pressure, and the presence of negative intrathoracic pressure facilitates the movement of fluid from the abdominal to pleural cavity through diaphragmatic defects leading to accumulation of fluid in the pleural space (3). Since the left diaphragm is thicker and more muscular than the right, nearly 80% of HH cases are seen on the right side (4). It should be noted that a significant number of HH cases are seen in the absence of any detectable ascites.

There was initial symptomatic improvement in breathlessness after aspiration. However, despite being on maximal doses of loop and potassium-sparing diuretics, there was a recurrence of the right pleural effusion (Figure 9.2).

b.  What non-pleural options are available in the management of hepatic hydrothorax?

Management of HH requires a multidisciplinary approach and is aimed at the reduction of ascites fluid formation, prevention of fluid transfer to the pleural space, removal and obliteration of the pleural space, and definitive management including liver transplantation. Sodium restriction (less than 2 g/day) and diuretics form the first line of management (5). Splanchnic and peripheral vasoconstrictors such as octreotide, midodrine and terlipressin have been occasionally used, and evidence is largely limited to case reports and series (6). Transjugular intrahepatic portosystemic shunt (TIPS), which aims to relieve portal hypertension, has response rates of nearly 70%–80% for HH. Continuous positive airway pressure (CPAP) therapy has been occasionally used, as it increases thoracic air pressure, decreasing the gradient between the pleural and peritoneal cavity and hence decreasing fluid movement into the pleural cavity. Surgical repair of diaphragmatic defects may be performed in select patients, however, it is usually avoided since it is associated with high morbidity and mortality (7).

Since the patient was in hepatic encephalopathy with an elevated MELD score, TIPS was contraindicated. The patient underwent a large volume thoracentesis where 1.5 litres of pleural fluid was aspirated.

c.  What pleural options are available in the treatment of hepatic hydrothorax?

Repeated thoracentesis can be performed in patients with refractory HH who are not candidates for TIPS or are awaiting a liver transplant; however, increasing numbers of procedures are associated with an increased risk of complications.

Chest tube drainage and pleurodesis is an option. However, retrospective studies have shown poorer outcomes than for malignant effusion, with increased mortality in this group possibly due to increased risk of empyema and sepsis (8). Tube thoracotomy is associated with significant hospital stays while awaiting pleurodesis.

Indwelling pleural catheters (IPCs) have been traditionally used in malignant pleural effusions and are associated with reduced hospital stay compared with talc pleurodesis. Their role has been extended to non-malignant pleural effusions; however, in a randomised trial by Walker et al. of transudative effusions, IPCs did not provide improved relief of dyspnoea when compared to repeated thoracentesis (9), even though IPCs drained about 17 litres and thoracentesis drained about 3 litres. There were more complications using IPCs, but it should be noted that not all the transudative effusions were related to HH (with some cardiac and renal failure patients).

IPCs in HH have recently gained momentum due to the lack of treatment options for non-transplantable patients. Most of the data stems from small and retrospective series. Spontaneous pleurodesis rates have been quoted to be about 30% in pure HH populations (2). In a retrospective review of 79 patients who underwent IPC placement for HH, pleural infection was seen in 8 (10%) patients and 2 (2.5%) patients died secondary to IPC-related sepsis (2). Hence, the decision to insert an IPC should be a multidisciplinary one including the transplant team and patient/carers, as IPCs are also associated with significant complications. IPCs may have a relevant role in non-transplantable patients, where symptom control and days out of hospital are the priority. However, in patients who are candidates for a liver transplant, IPCs should be inserted with caution, as IPC-related pleural infection may preclude a transplant (10). In our practice, if a patient requires more than three thoracentesis for symptom relief, we discuss IPC treatment if a transplant and TIPS are not options.

After 2 weeks, it was noted that the HH had re-accumulated. Since she was not a candidate for a liver transplant, a decision was made to insert an IPC to relieve her dyspnoea. The patient had deranged clotting and was consented for additional bleeding risk. The IPC was inserted with no complications (Figure 9.3) and she was discharged with a drainage strategy up to three times per week. Following the insertion, the patient complained of IPC leakage with excoriation of the surrounding skin. Therefore, two sutures were

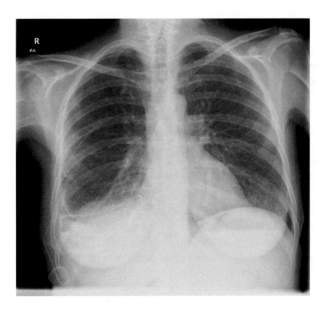

Figure 9.3 Chest X-ray after insertion of IPC.

inserted to tighten the tract and an aggressive drainage strategy (800–1000 ml every day for 3 weeks) was adopted to try to achieve pleurodesis. After 3 weeks, an ultrasound of the right side revealed minimal fluid, IPC in situ and minimal lung sliding, indicating likely auto-pleurodesis. Therefore, a decision was made to remove the IPC. On follow-up after 1 month, there were no signs of fluid re-accumulation.

## KEY POINTS

- A liver transplant is the definitive treatment for refractory HH.
- Repeated thoracentesis may be an option for patients waiting for liver transplantation.
- IPC has a role in patients who are not liver transplant candidates, desire home treatment or in those where stoppage of anticoagulation is unfavourable.
- IPC-related pleural infection remains a serious problem in this cohort.

## REFERENCES

1. Hung TH, Tseng CW, Tsai CC, Tsai CC, Tseng KC, Hsieh YH. The long-term outcomes of cirrhotic patients with pleural effusion. *Saudi J Gastroenterol* 2018;24(1):46–51.
2. Shojaee S, Rahman N, Haas K, et al. Indwelling tunneled pleural catheters for refractory hepatic hydrothorax in patients with cirrhosis: A multi-center study. *Chest* 2019;155(3):546–553.
3. Huang PM, Chang YL, Yang CY, Lee YC. The morphology of diaphragmatic defects in hepatic hydrothorax: Thoracoscopic finding. *J Thorac Cardiovasc Surg* 2005;130(1):141–145.
4. Gurung P, Goldblatt M, Huggins JT, Doelken P, Nietert PJ, Sahn SA. Pleural fluid analysis and radiographic, sonographic, and echocardiographic characteristics of hepatic hydrothorax. *Chest* 2011;140(2):448–453.
5. Runyon BA; AASLD. Introduction to the revised American Association for the Study of Liver Diseases Practice Guideline management of adult patients with ascites due to cirrhosis 2012. *Hepatology* 2013;57(4):1651–1653.
6. Runyon BA. Management of adult patients with ascites due to cirrhosis. *Hepatology* 2004;39(3):841–856.
7. Banini BA, Alwatari Y, Stovall M, et al. Multidisciplinary management of hepatic hydrothorax in 2020: An evidence-based review and guidance. *Hepatology* 2020;72(5):1851–1863.

8. Hung TH, Tseng CW, Tsai CC, et al. Mortality following catheter drainage versus thoracentesis in cirrhotic patients with pleural effusion. *Dig Dis Sci* 2017;62(4):1080–1085.
9. Walker SP, Bintcliffe O, Keenan E, et al. Randomised trial of indwelling pleural catheters for refractory transudative pleural effusions. *Eur Respir J* 2022;59(2):2101362.
10. Gilbert CR, Shojaee S, Maldonado F, et al. Pleural interventions in the management of hepatic hydrothorax. *Chest* 2022;161(1):276–283.

# 10

# Pleural effusion and thickening after asbestos exposure

HUI GUO

A 67-year-old retired builder presented to hospital with progressive dyspnoea and a large, left-sided pleural effusion. His medical history was significant for atypical chronic myelogenous leukaemia (CML) in remission after a sibling allograft bone marrow transplant, complicated by cutaneous, ocular and pulmonary graft versus host disease. His regular medications were cyclosporin, penicillin V, co-trimoxazole, acyclovir, azithromycin and entecavir. He was managed for asthma with regular inhaled budesonide and as-needed salbutamol. He had asbestos exposure in his previous occupation and was an ex-smoker of <10 pack-years.

He reported months of recurrent respiratory infections receiving multiple courses of oral antibiotics in the community.

He underwent ultrasound-guided thoracocentesis (Figures 10.1–10.3). Pleural biochemistry demonstrated protein 41 g/L, glucose 6.2 mmol/L and LDH 320 IU/L. Pleural fluid microbiology was negative, and cytology demonstrated blood and scattered inflammatory cells. Chest X-rays were performed before and after the procedure.

a) What is the differential diagnosis?

Pleural malignancy is the most likely diagnosis, given the history of immunosuppression, lack of response to antibiotics and asbestos exposure (as evidenced by both history and pleural plaques on chest X-ray). The appearance of the post-procedure X-ray demonstrating left-sided hydropneumothorax and likely trapped lung infers potential pleural thickening, which suggests potential malignancy.

The ultrasonographic appearance of the fluid is echogenic and free flowing without septations. The pleural fluid is mildly inflammatory with normal

DOI: 10.1201/9781003081630-10

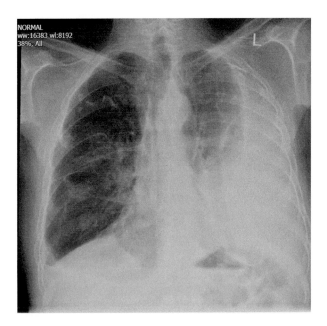

Figure 10.1 Chest X-ray showing left-sided pleural effusion.

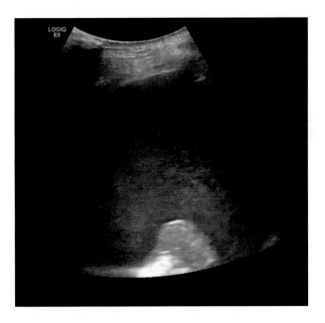

Figure 10.2 Left-sided ultrasound image showing echogenic pleural effusion.

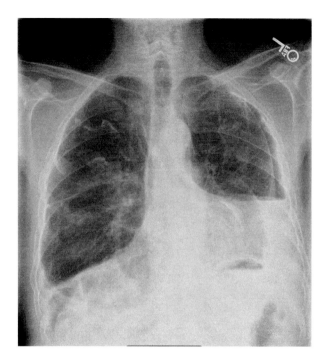

Figure 10.3 Chest X-ray post-pleural aspiration showing left-sided hydropneumothorax.

glucose. Both point away from a complicated parapneumonic effusion or empyema. It is worth noting, however, that negative microbiology in general does not exclude pleural infection. In the landmark MIST1 trial of 454 patients with pleural infection, about 40% were gram stain and culture negative (1).

Similarly, the lack of malignant cells on cytology does not exclude malignancy. A meta-analysis of 36 studies including 6,057 patients determined the overall sensitivity of pleural fluid cytology to be 58% for diagnosing malignancy (2), with variability between tumour types.

As the CML is in remission, it is unlikely that the effusion is related to direct leukaemic infiltration. Graft versus host disease can manifest with serositis-related pleural effusions, however, this is rare (3).

The patient proceeded to a pleural biopsy via medical thoracoscopy. On macroscopic inspection (Figure 10.4), there were multiple pleural plaques and diffuse inflammation with lymphangitis over the parietal, visceral and diaphragmatic surfaces. No discrete nodularity was seen.

The pleura histopathology demonstrated fibrosis with mild chronic inflammation without evidence of lymphoma or mesothelial malignancy, but with no fat identified in the biopsies.

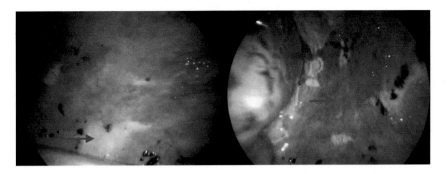

Figure 10.4 Macroscopic appearance on thoracoscopy showing diffuse plaques (red arrow) with lymphangitis (blue arrow).

b) What is the role of medical thoracoscopy in evaluating undifferentiated pleural effusions?

Medical thoracoscopy is the procedure of choice in investigating a unilateral exudative pleural effusion with non-diagnostic pleural cytology (4). It has a high sensitivity (93%) in diagnosing malignancy (5), and allows for simultaneous talc poudrage pleurodesis and/or insertion of an intrapleural catheter (IPC). This combines high diagnostic yield with definitive pleural fluid management in a population where symptomatic effusion is likely to recur. Medical thoracoscopy is safe with a mortality rate of 0.34% on combined data from 47 studies (5), with mortality largely attributable to the use of non-graded talc from USA studies (6). The mortality directly attributable to diagnostic thoracoscopy is close to 0%.

Given the high clinical suspicion of malignancy and recurrence of pleural effusion, a repeat left-sided thoracoscopy was performed 1 month later with the addition of a cutting needle biopsy, providing out-to-in biopsy samples and enabling assessment of the underlying fat. Histology once again showed benign fibrosis without malignancy with fat represented in the pleural biopsy.

A macroscopic view on thoracoscopy confirmed the previous chest X-ray findings of trapped lung, and the decision was made to insert an IPC post-thoracoscopy instead of using talc poudrage.

A thoracic CT was performed prior to the second thoracoscopy (Figure 10.5).

c) What does the CT show? What is the most likely diagnosis?

Mediastinal windows of the CT Figure 10.5) show bilateral pleural plaques (blue arrows) with left-sided visceral pleural thickening (red arrow), reinforced by the presence of pleuroparenchymal bands (green arrow). The latter is more clearly demonstrated on the lung windows. There is a degree of mosaicism in the lung parenchyma, consistent with known asthma and small airways disease.

With two negative biopsies for malignancy and a suggestive exposure history, the most likely diagnosis here is benign asbestos pleural effusion

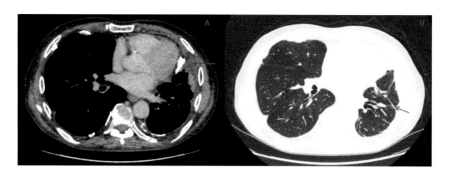

Figure 10.5 (A) Mediastinal and (B) lung window of thoracic CT.

(BAPE). This forms part of the spectrum of asbestos-related pleural diseases, consisting of pleural plaque, diffuse pleural thickening and malignant pleural mesothelioma. BAPE is diagnosed in individuals with known asbestos exposure for whom other causes of pleural effusion, especially malignancy, have been excluded (hence the importance of a pleural biopsy). The American Thoracic Society recommends a follow-up period of 3 years before the pleural effusion is definitively labelled benign (7).

BAPE typically manifests 10–20 years after asbestos exposure (8) and tends to resolve spontaneously (9), although it can recur ipsilaterally or contralaterally (10). The effusion is exudative, often haemorrhagic and the cytology usually consists of mixed inflammatory cells or predominantly eosinophils (11,12). There is no current evidence to suggest that BAPE develops into malignant pleural mesothelioma, however, the shared risk factor (asbestos exposure) for both conditions should be noted.

The left-sided IPC continued to drain 200 ml twice a week and a 3-month interval thoracic CT demonstrated radiological stability of the left-sided pleural thickening.

Unfortunately, 5 months later, he presented to haematology clinic again feeling dyspnoeic. Thoracic CT was performed and showed a new right (contralateral)-sided pleural effusion. This was aspirated and demonstrated similar exudative biochemistry to the left-sided effusion, with protein 35 g/L, glucose 6.5 mmol/L and LDH 361 IU/L. Microbiology was negative and cytology was mostly blood.

After multidisciplinary discussion, plans were made to conduct a medical thoracoscopy on the right, following the same diagnostic pathway as for the left. Sadly, during this time, the CML relapsed and he passed away shortly after.

## KEY POINTS

- Benign asbestos pleural effusion (BAPE) is a diagnosis of exclusion.
- The entity presents very similarly to malignant effusion and mesothelioma in asbestos-exposed individuals with a usually blood-stained effusion.

- Where possible, pleural biopsy (ideally thoracoscopic or surgical) should be undertaken to thoroughly exclude malignant pleural disease.
- Management is in general supportive and can require strategies for pleural fluid control.

## REFERENCES

1. Maskell NA, Davies CW, Nunn AJ, et al. U.K. Controlled trial of intrapleural streptokinase for pleural infection. *N Engl J Med* 2005;352(9):865–874.
2. Kassirian S, Hinton SN, Cuninghame S, et al. Diagnostic sensitivity of pleural fluid cytology in malignant pleural effusions: systematic review and meta-analysis. *Thorax.* 2023;78(1):32–40.
3. Modi D, Jang H, Kim S, et al. Incidence, etiology, and outcome of pleural effusions in allogeneic hematopoietic stem cell transplantation. *Am J Hematol* 2016;91(9):E341–E347.
4. Hooper C, Lee YC, Maskell N, BTS Pleural Guideline Group. Investigation of a unilateral pleural effusion in adults: British Thoracic Society pleural disease guideline 2010. *Thorax* 2010;65;Suppl 2:ii4–ii17.
5. Rahman NM, Ali NJ, Brown G, et al. Local anaesthetic thoracoscopy: British Thoracic Society pleural disease guideline 2010. *Thorax* 2010;65;Suppl 2:ii54–ii60.
6. Dresler CM, Olak J, Herndon 2nd JE, et al. Phase III intergroup study of talc poudrage vs talc slurry sclerosis for malignant pleural effusion. *Chest* 2005;127(3):909–915.
7. American Thoracic Society. Diagnosis and initial management of non-malignant diseases related to asbestos. *Am J Respir Crit Care Med* 2004;170(6):691–715.
8. Cookson WO, De Klerk NH, Musk AW, Glancy JJ, Armstrong BK, Hobbs MS. Benign and malignant pleural effusions in former Wittenoom crocidolite millers and miners. *Aust N Z J Med* 1985;15(6):731–737.
9. Musk AW, de Klerk N, Reid A, Hui J, Franklin P, Brims F. Asbestos-related diseases. *Int J Tuberc Lung Dis* 2020;24(6):562–567.
10. Myers R. Asbestos-related pleural disease. *Curr Opin Pulm Med* 2012;18(4):377–381.
11. Fujimoto N, Gemba K, Aoe K, et al. Clinical investigation of benign asbestos pleural effusion. *Pulm Med* 2015;2015:416179.
12. Hillerdal G, Ozesmi M. Benign asbestos pleural effusion: 73 exudates in 60 patients. *Eur J Respir Dis* 1987;71(2):113–121.

# 11

# Recurrent effusion in a cyclist

## DINESH ADDALA

A 61-year-old male presented to the pleural service with breathlessness, fatigue and no other constitutional symptoms. He was an employee in a technology firm, never smoked and reported exercising regularly. He had previously been investigated for unilateral pleural effusion 6 years prior, which had resolved with aspiration only.

His CT scan on presentation is demonstrated in Figure 11.1.

a) What are the features illustrated on the CT scan in Figure 11.1?

The CT scan illustrates a moderate left-sided pleural effusion, with parenchymal ground glass opacification ipsilateral to the pleural effusion. The right side demonstrates appearances consistent with rounded atelectasis. The cardiac size appears normal.

b) What is the best modality of CT scan to undertake for the diagnosis of pleural disease?

To detect pleural pathology, intravenous contrast, (late venous phase) with the scan occurring 60–90 seconds after contrast injection is recommended (1,2), especially for identification of typical malignant features, which are usually the most common cause.

c) Should the patient have their pleural fluid drained prior to a CT scan?

In the detection of pleural-based pathology, it is recommended to leave fluid in the patient to accentuate the difference in density between pleura and fluid. Lung masses, when present, are generally not compressible by fluid and thus retain their structure even in the presence of a large pleural effusion (1). Small pulmonary nodules may be obscured by large pleural effusions, but this has not been shown to occur frequently in a specific study designed to address this.

The patient went on to undergo basic blood tests, and a diagnostic and therapeutic pleural aspiration of the left-sided pleural effusion. An example of thoracic

DOI: 10.1201/9781003081630-11

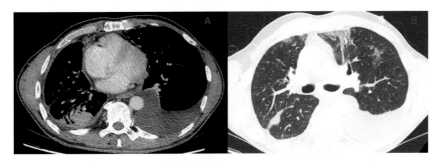

Figure 11.1 (A) Mediastinal and (B) lung window of thoracic CT.

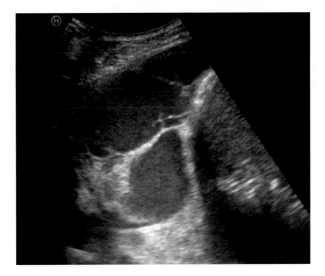

Figure 11.2 Left-sided thoracic ultrasound showing the presence of moderately sized, densely echogenic and septated effusion.

ultrasound peri-procedurally demonstrated densely echogenic pleural effusion, moderate in size and with early septations as shown in Figure 11.2.

The blood and pleural fluid results are as follows:

*Blood*: Hb 113 g/L, WCC 5190/mm$^3$, neutrophils 3710/mm$^3$, lymphocytes 600/mm$^3$, CRP 20 g/L

*Pleural fluid*: protein 50g/dL, LDH 174 IU/L, glucose 5.6 mmol/L, cholesterol 2.2 mmol/L, triglycerides 37.95 mmol/L; chylomicrons present, no cholesterol crystals

d) What type of pleural effusion does the pleural fluid indicate?

The pleural fluid indicates that this is a chylothorax. Table 11.1 indicates the key pleural fluid characteristics that distinguish chylothorax from

Table 11.1 Biochemical features of chylothorax and pseudochylothorax (3)

| Feature | Pseudochylothorax | Chylothorax |
|---|---|---|
| Triglycerides | | >1.24 mml/L (110 mg/dL) |
| Cholesterol | >5.18 mmol/L (200 mg/dL) | Low |
| Cholesterol crystals | Often present | Absent |
| Chylomicrons | Absent | Usually present |

pseudochylothorax. Macroscopically, chylothorax is often described as 'milky' in appearance.

e) What are the common causes of chylothorax?

Common causes of chylothorax include trauma, neoplasm, lymphatic disorders and idiopathic (approximately 10%). Non-traumatic causes of chylous effusion account for 25%–50% of cases (4).

The most common causes of pseudochylothorax include tuberculosis and rheumatoid arthritis.

He went on to suffer repeated pleural effusions requiring drainage on the left side, with a small right pleural effusion. He reported that symptoms of breathlessness and accumulation of pleural effusion appeared to be related to extensive exercise. He went on to undergo a pleural biopsy of the left, which showed inflammation only and did not identify an obvious cause of recurrent chylothorax.

f) What further imaging tests are available to help with achieving a diagnosis?

In cases of challenging-to-diagnose chylothorax, with no known underlying malignant or systemic cause, an MRI lymphangiogram (5) can be used to assess the possibility of a thoracic duct leak or anatomical abnormality leading to pleural effusion or chylothorax formation. Other options include conventional lymphography (injection of methylene blue and monitoring on serial radiographs), which is invasive, time-consuming and rarely conducted as part of routine clinical practice. Additionally, SPECT-CT (nuclear medicine) can associate anatomical and functional imaging and can identify diffuse lymphatic disease or lymphatic leak, but again require ionising radiation and specialist resources (5).

The results of his MRI lymphangiogram are illustrated in Figure 11.3.

The MRI showed contrast opacification along the left para-aortic lymphatic chain with the cisterna chyli demonstrated at the level of the diaphragm (T11/T12), an enhancing fluid collection in the middle mediastinum (labelled by the white arrow), which appears to communicate with the thoracic duct. Enhancing fluid was noted to track into the right pleural effusion (labelled with a blue arrow) along the bronchovascular bundles. A small increase in left basal effusion was demonstrated (labelled by the star).

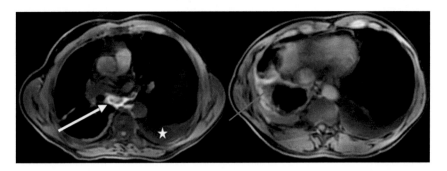

Figure 11.3 MRI lymphangiogram depicting lymphatic vessels and thorax.

Overall, the images were consistent with a lymphatic leak into the right pleural effusion from the thoracic duct. The scan demonstrated that at the level of the thoracic duct disruption, leakage into the left pleural space would be expected but was not demonstrated.

Over the course of the following months, the patient experienced deteriorating breathlessness, and despite a good performance status, his exercise tolerance declined despite intermittent pleural aspiration. He developed pleural thickening and his lung function deteriorated significantly with a restrictive deficit.

g) What further options are available for management?

Key steps in the management of chylothorax include a low-fat diet, specifically low in long-chain fatty acids, which are used to form chyle. Medium- and short-chain triglycerides are absorbed into the portal system, bypassing the intestinal lymph system and reducing the flow of chyle in the thoracic duct (6).

Other options for the management of chylothorax include alpha-1 adrenergic agonists such as midodrine (7), which cause vasoconstriction of the lymph system, but can result in the side effects of headaches and urinary frequency. The somatostatin analogue octreotide has also been used in specific cases (mostly post-operative), inhibiting gastric pancreatic and biliary secretions, and inhibiting chyle resorption from the intestines (8).

The aforementioned options were all trialled with limited benefits and side effects.

This patient was of a good performance status with progressive pleural thickening and worsening lung function with symptoms. He was refractory to medical management; it would be appropriate to consider surgical intervention here. In this case, due to the presence of pleural thickening (beyond recurrent chylothorax), lung release pleurectomy and thoracic duct ligation was undertaken. In cases of recurrent chylothorax only, thoracic duct embolisation or pleurodesis can be considered (9).

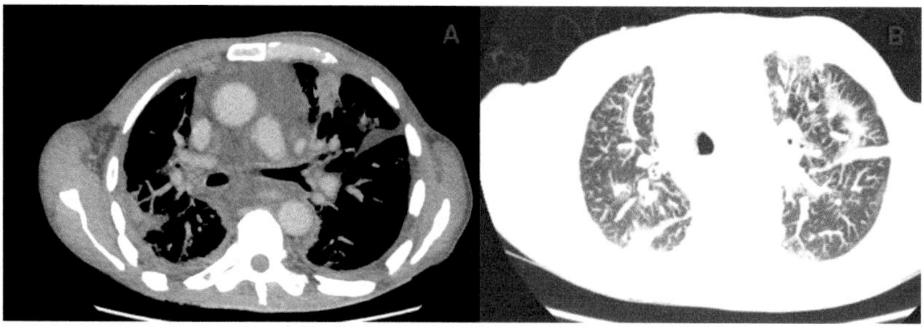

Figure 11.4 (A) Mediastinal and (B) lung window of thoracic CT.

The patient underwent a challenging clinical course post-surgery with only transient improvement in symptoms. He, unfortunately, experienced recurrent chylothorax complicated by pleural infection, requiring a further ipsilateral video-assisted thoracoscopy for decortication and washout.

His subsequent medium-term recovery was complicated by hypercapnic respiratory failure, which raised the possibility of lung parenchymal involvement (hypercapnic failure can be seen in bilateral pleural disease but is unusual in the absence of a further contributory cause such as lung parenchymal disease, upper airway disease or muscular weakness). His CT scans at this stage are illustrated in Figure 11.4.

The CT scans show significant mediastinal enlargement and intralobular septal thickening which had progressed markedly. Rib crowding is demonstrated and there are large intrapulmonary nodules. These changes were thought by consensus at multidisciplinary team meetings to represent diffuse lymphangiomatosis.

Diffuse lymphangiomatosis can present in a range of ways, with multiple organs affected. Chylothorax, pericardial effusions and bone involvement have been reported. The pathophysiology is due to progressive lymphatic vessel proliferation of unknown causes.

Specific treatment of this condition is limited to case series and case reports, however, bevacizumab and sirolimus have been reported in the literature to have been used with success (10,11).

Unfortunately, this patient was not well enough to tolerate these treatments and required symptom-based control and ventilatory support.

## KEY POINTS

- Chylothorax has specific biochemical features, and although the diagnosis is usually suggested by the macroscopic appearances, these are not always present.
- The diagnosis of chylothorax needs careful consideration of the underlying cause – investigation will usually require a thoracic CT scan and may require lymphatic radiological assessment.

- Treatment is best directed at the underlying cause, including establishing if there is a single leak in the thoracic duct (and therefore amenable to surgical or ablation therapy) or diffuse abnormalities, which require systemic treatment or pleurodesis.
- Treatments directed at reducing dietary fat or reducing splanchnic blood flow (somatostatin analogues or midodrine) can be helpful.

## REFERENCES

1. Corcoran JP, Acton L, Ahmed A, Hallifax RJ, Psallidas I, Wrightson JM, Rahman NM, Gleeson FV. Diagnostic value of radiological imaging pre- and post-drainage of pleural effusions. *Respirology.* 2016 February;21(2):392–395.
2. Arenas-Jiménez JJ, García-Garrigós E, Escudero-Fresneda C, et al. Early and delayed phases of contrast-enhanced CT for evaluating patients with malignant pleural effusion. Results of pairwise comparison by multiple observers. *British Journal of Radiology.* 2018;91(1089):20180254.
3. Rudrappa M, Paul M. Chylothorax [Updated 2023 Feb 21]. In: *StatPearls.* [Internet]. Treasure Island (FL): StatPearls Publishing. 2023. Jan. Available from: https://www.ncbi.nlm.nih.gov/books/NBK459206/
4. Gurevich A, Hur S, Singhal S, et al. Nontraumatic chylothorax and chylopericardium: Diagnosis and treatment using an algorithmic approach based on novel lymphatic imaging. *Annals ATS.* 2022;19(5):756–762.
5. Cholet C, Delalandre C, Monnier-Cholley L, Le Pimpec-Barthes F, El Mouhadi S, Arrivé L. Nontraumatic chylothorax: Nonenhanced MR lymphography. *RadioGraphics.* 2020;40(6):1554–1573.
6. McGrath EE, Blades Z, Anderson PB. Chylothorax: Aetiology, diagnosis and therapeutic options. *Respiratory Medicine.* 2010;104(1):1–8.
7. Liou DZ, Warren H, Maher DP, et al. Midodrine: A novel therapeutic for refractory chylothorax. *Chest.* 2013;144(3):1055–1057.
8. Sharkey AJ, Rao JN. The successful use of octreotide in the treatment of traumatic chylothorax. *Texas Heart Institute Journal.* 2012;39(3):428–430.
9. Iqbal B, Rahman NM. Chyle in the wrong place: Why knowing the target matters. *Annals ATS.* 2022;19(5):722–723.
10. Onyeforo E, Barnett A, Zagami D, Deller D, Feather I. Diffuse pulmonary lymphangiomatosis treated with bevacizumab. *Respirology Case Reports.* 2018;7(1):e00384.
11. Ozeki M, Nozawa A, Yasue S, et al. The impact of sirolimus therapy on lesion size, clinical symptoms, and quality of life of patients with lymphatic anomalies. *Orphanet Journal of Rare Diseases.* 2019;14(1):141.

# 12

# Pleural thickening and effusion in a traveller

HUI GUO

A 70-year-old man with chronic lymphocytic leukaemia (CLL) in remission on ibrutinib for the last 4.5 years presented to his haematologist with a lesion on his left forearm and 5 months of cough. Other past medical history entries included bladder polyps, which were non-malignant on biopsy. He was not taking any other medications except ibrutinib. He was a retired company board member and previously also worked as an accountant. Post-retirement, he lived on a farm with sheep. He was a current smoker of 15 cigarettes per day. Of note, he frequently travelled to Mexico and Malta.

The forearm lesion appeared 4 to 5 months prior to presentation and was static during that time. From time to time it formed a crust (Figure 12.1). The cough began shortly after he received the flu vaccination 5 months ago and was associated with left-sided chest discomfort, anorexia and weight loss. There was no history of fevers or sweats.

Biopsy of this lesion was undertaken and demonstrated granulomatous dermatitis. The *Leishmania donovani* PCR was positive. Fungal and mycobacterial cultures were negative.

A chest X-ray was performed to investigate the cough and demonstrated a left-sided pleural effusion which was new compared to his lymphoma staging CT scan 4 months prior (Figure 12.2).

A pleural ultrasound (US) revealed a large, free-flowing, non-echogenic effusion with associated basal atelectasis and a normally shaped but sluggishly moving diaphragm (Figure 12.3).

The pleural effusion was aspirated with 1000 ml drained under ultrasound guidance. Biochemistry showed protein 43 g/L, glucose 5.2 mmol/L and LDH 253 IU/L.

DOI: 10.1201/9781003081630-12

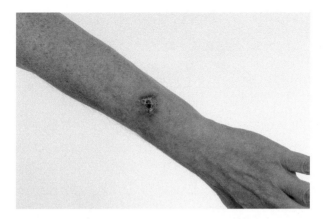

Figure 12.1 Nodular ulcerated lesion with scab formation on left forearm.

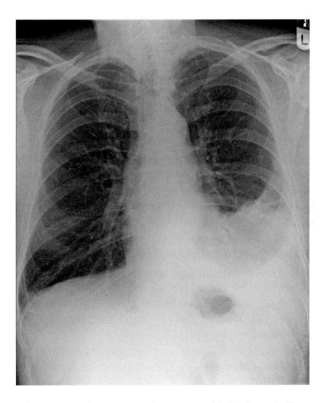

Figure 12.2 Chest X-ray showing moderate-sized left pleural effusion.

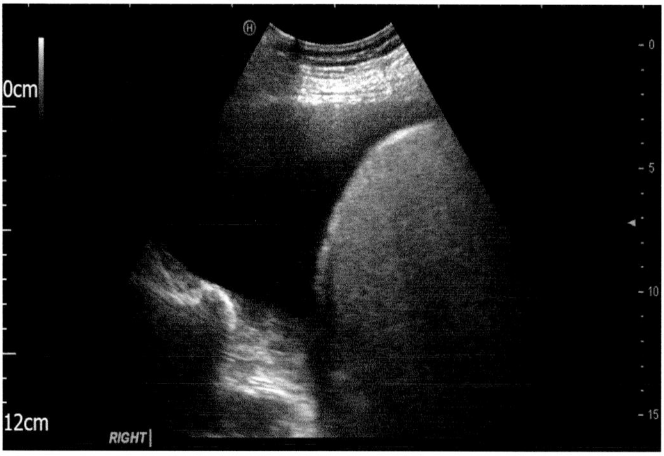

Figure 12.3 Left-sided US image showing left pleural effusion.

Fluid cytology contained blood, benign mesothelial cells, some neutrophils and moderate numbers of small lymphocytes. On immunocytochemistry, the lymphocytes were almost exclusively CD3/CD5+ T cells, with only very occasional CD20/CD79a+ B cells, in keeping with a reactive effusion.

He was planned for intralesional injections of stibogluconate to manage the cutaneous leishmaniasis, however, this was not yet commenced at the time of the pleural aspiration.

a) What is the differential diagnosis for this pleural effusion?

Unilateral pleural effusion in an immunosuppressed smoker with known haematological malignancy raises suspicion for both malignancy and infection. The pleural fluid is a mildly inflammatory exudate which could be in keeping with both these diagnoses.

CLL can cause pleural effusions through various mechanisms: (a) direct leukaemic infiltration; (b) lymphatic obstruction causing chylothorax; and (c) drug-related effusions, including tyrosine kinase inhibitors (TKI) such as ibrutinib (1). For this patient, who has been in remission and stable on ibrutinib for many years, all these possibilities are unlikely. However, a separate malignancy such as lung or pleural, especially given the smoking history, should be considered.

The travel history and subacute course of illness suggest atypical infection such as tuberculosis. The lymphocytic predominant cytology would be in keeping with this, although lower glucose might be expected with this degree of symptom chronicity. Pleural fluid culture has a variable sensitivity of 12%–70% (2) in diagnosing tuberculous pleuritis, with a yield of up to 79% (3) when combined with pleural biopsy.

Finally, *Leishmania donovani* infection itself can manifest with pleural effusions in rare instances, usually in the immunosuppressed patient (4–6).

Post-aspiration, he underwent a repeat thoracic ultrasound and thoracic CT, which are shown in Figures 12.4 and 12.5.

b) What do the thoracic ultrasound and CT scan show?

The thoracic ultrasound shows a small heavily septated effusion with parietal and visceral pleural thickening.

The CT scan shows a left pleural effusion with the 'split pleura sign' (arrow) with smooth enhancement of both the visceral and parietal pleura with pleural thickening adjacent to the aorta and nodularity over the mediastinum.

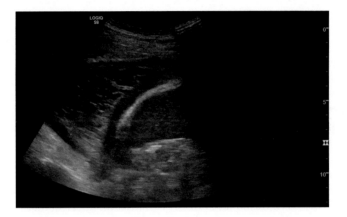

Figure 12.4 Post-aspiration US image.

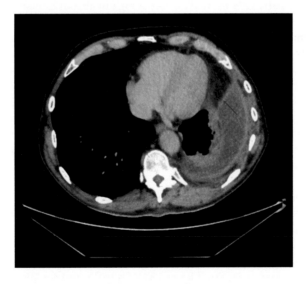

Figure 12.5 Mediastinal window of thoracic CT scan.

c) What are the differential diagnoses for the pleural thickening? What features are concerning and how should they be investigated?

Pleural thickening in this case could relate either to malignancy or chronic infection.

Features suggestive of malignant pleural thickening are (a) circumferential thickening, (b) pleural nodularity, (c) parietal thickening >1 cm and (d) mediastinal involvement. In small cohort studies (7–8), these features have been demonstrated to have sensitivity of 72%–84% and specificity of 83%–100% in differentiating benign from malignant pleural disease. The largest retrospective study of 211 patients (9) correlating 'malignant' appearing CT to thoracoscopic biopsy results demonstrated a sensitivity of 68% and specificity of 78% for CT imaging in predicting pleural malignancy.

Features on CT that favour infection over malignancy are (a) lentiform (bi-convex) effusion, (b) visceral pleural thickening with the 'split pleura sign', (c) extrapleural fat hypertrophy, (d) increased density of extrapleural fat and (e) lung consolidation. These features are highly specific (85%–97%) but poorly sensitive (20%–37% (10–11) and certainly infection and malignancy can co-exist.

In the absence of a unifying diagnosis and persistence of a unilateral pleural effusion, the next investigative step would be to perform a pleural biopsy.

d) How should the pleural biopsy be obtained?

The most sensitive methods for obtaining pleural biopsy are via image guidance (CT or ultrasound) or direct visualisation (medical thoracoscopy or video-assisted thoracic surgery [VATS]). These targeted procedures have largely replaced the traditional 'blind' pleural biopsy.

The diagnostic yield for malignancy is high in all four modalities. For image-guided biopsies, reported sensitivities range from 70% to 94% (12–18), and are comparable between ultrasound and CT (19). Pooled data from 22 case series demonstrates a sensitivity of 93% for medical thoracoscopy (20). Whilst there have been no direct comparisons, this is similar to the sensitivity of VATS pleural biopsy (95%) (21). Both medical thoracoscopy and VATS allow for simultaneous therapeutic options (e.g. pleurodesis) and have good safety profiles.

Other practical considerations include the patient's general performance status, tolerance of the lateral decubitus position, location of pleural thickening, accessibility of pleural space and service availability.

The patient proceeded to pleural biopsy via medical thoracoscopy, however, on pre-procedure ultrasound, the pleural space was heavily septated with sluggish lung sliding above and hence difficult to access via thoracoscope. Instead, ultrasound-guided pleural biopsies were undertaken.

The histopathology results showed necrotising granulomatous inflammation favouring infectious aetiology (Figure 12.6). Special stains for leishmanias, fungal organisms and mycobacteria were negative.

At this time, the patient completed a course of intralesional stibogluconate for his cutaneous leishmaniasis. His repeat thoracic CT performed 3 months later demonstrated interval improvement of his left-sided pleural collection and thickening (Figure 12.7).

The diagnosis for his pleural effusion was concluded to be related to leishmaniasis, given regression on treatment.

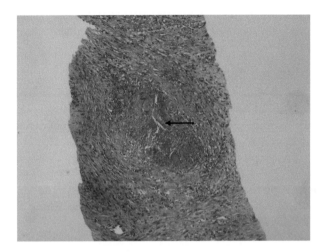

Figure 12.6 Haematoxylin and eosin stain of the parietal pleura showing the presence of necrotising granulomatous inflammation (black arrow).

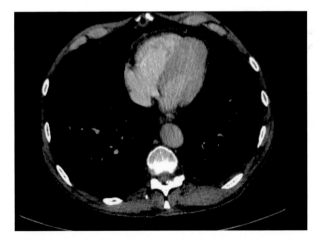

Figure 12.7 Mediastinal window of thoracic CT scan.

## KEY POINTS

- Inflammatory pleural effusions on radiology and biochemistry retain a wide differential diagnosis, and either pleural malignancy or infection (acute and chronic) should be suspected.
- Pleural biopsy remains a valuable tool in the differentiation of these entities and allows exclusion of pleural malignancy.
- CT thorax findings have potentially distinct characteristics comparing malignant and chronic infectious pleural diseases, but no features are 100% sensitive or specific.

## REFERENCES

1. Styskel BA, Lopez-Mattei J, Jimenez CA, Stewart J, Hagemeister FB, Faiz SA. Ibrutinib-associated serositis in mantle cell lymphoma. *Am J Respir Crit Care Med.* 2019;199(12):e43–e44.
2. Sibley JC. A study of 200 cases of tuberculous pleurisy with effusion. *Am Rev Tuberc.* 1950;62(3):314.e23.
3. Diacon AH, Van de Wal BW, Wyser C, et al. Diagnostic tools in tuberculous pleurisy: A direct comparative study. *Eur Respir J.* 2003;22(4):589–591.
4. Chenoweth CE, Singal S, Pearson RD, Betts RF, Markovitz DM. Acquired immunodeficiency syndrome-related visceral leishmaniasis presenting in a pleural effusion. *Chest.* 1993;103(2):648–649.
5. Das VN, Pandey K, Kumar N, Hassan SM, Bimal S, Lal CS, et al. Visceral leishmaniasis and tuberculosis in patients with HIV co-infection. *Southeast Asian J Trop Med Public Health.* 2006;37(1):18–21.
6. Diehl RS, Santos RP, Zimmerman R, Luz LP, Weiss T, Jacobson P, et al. Microscopy and polymerase chain reaction detection of *Leishmania chagasi* in the pleural and ascitic fluid of a patient with AIDS: Case report and review of diagnosis and therapy of visceral leishmaniasis. *Can J Infect Dis Med Microbiol.* 2004;15(4):231–234.
7. Leung AN, Müller NL, Miller RR. CT in differential diagnosis of diffuse pleural disease. *AJR Am J Roentgenol.* 1990;154(3):487–492.
8. Traill ZC, Davies RJO, Gleeson FV. Thoracic computed tomography in patients with suspected malignant pleural effusions. *Clin Radiol.* 2001 March;56(3):193–196.
9. Hallifax RJ, Haris M, Corcoran JP, Leyakathalikhan S, Brown E, Srikantharaja D, et al. Role of CT in assessing pleural malignancy prior to thoracoscopy. *Thorax.* 2014 July 30;70(2):192–193.
10. Arenas-Jimenez J, Alonso-Charterina S, Sanchez-Paya J, Fernandez-Latorre F, Gil-Sanchez S, Lloret-Llorens M. Evaluation of CT findings for diagnosis of pleural effusions. *Eur Radiol.* 2000;10(4):681–690.

11. Yilmaz U, Polat G, Sahin N, Soy O, Gülay U. CT in differential diagnosis of benign and malignant pleural disease. *Monaldi Arch Chest Dis.* 2005;63(1):17–22.
12. Maskell NA, Gleeson FV, Davies RJ. Standard pleural biopsy versus CT-guided cutting-needle biopsy for diagnosis of malignant disease in pleural effusions: A randomised controlled trial. *Lancet.* 2003;361(9366):1326–1330.
13. Chang DB, Yang PC, Luh KT, Kuo SH, Yu CJ. Ultrasound-guided pleural biopsy with Tru-Cut needle. *Chest.* 1991;100(5):1328–1333.
14. Adams RF, Gray W, Davies RJ, Gleeson FV. Percutaneous image-guided cutting needle biopsy of the pleura in the diagnosis of malignant mesothelioma. *Chest.* 2001;120(6):1798–1802.
15. Benamore RE, Scott K, Richards CJ, Entwisle JJ. Image-guided pleural biopsy: Diagnostic yield and complications. *Clin Radiol.* 2006;61(8):700–705.
16. Scott EM, Marshall TJ, Flower CD, Stewart S. Diffuse pleural thickening: Percutaneous CT-guided cutting needle biopsy. *Radiology.* 1995;194(3):867–870.
17. Metintaş M, Ozdemir N, Işiksoy S, et al. CT-guided pleural needle biopsy in the diagnosis of malignant mesothelioma. *J Comput Assist Tomogr.* 1995;19(3):370–374.
18. Mueller PR, Saini S, Simeone JF, et al. Image-guided pleural biopsies: Indications, technique, and results in 23 patients. *Radiology.* 1988;169(1):1–4.
19. Sconfienza LM, Mauri G, Grossi F, et al. Pleural and peripheral lung lesions: Comparison of US- and CT-guided biopsy. *Radiology.* 2013;266(3):930–935.
20. Rahman NM, Ali NJ, Brown G, et al. Local anaesthetic thoracoscopy: British Thoracic Society Pleural Disease Guideline 2010. *Thorax.* 2010;65;Suppl 2:ii54–ii60.
21. Hooper C, Lee YC, Maskell N, et al. BTS Pleural Guideline Group. Investigation of a unilateral pleural effusion in adults: British Thoracic Society Pleural Disease Guideline 2010. *Thorax.* 2010;65;Suppl 2:ii4–ii17.

# 13

# Recurrent effusion in a patient on amiodarone

## NAJIB M RAHMAN

A 78-year-old woman presented to the pleural clinic with a history of admission for respiratory infection one month earlier. She had been treated as an inpatient for pneumonia based on raised inflammatory markers and some right-sided lung infiltrate but had required three episodes of antibiotics. A CT pulmonary angiogram was performed by the admitting team during admission, which demonstrated a right basal effusion, basal consolidation and no evidence of pulmonary embolus. She presented 1 month later with breathlessness.

Her past history included colon cancer treated with curative intent (hemicolectomy) 15 years ago, atrial fibrillation and asthma, and she was treated with amiodarone (for the last 10 years), inhaled ICS/LABA and apixaban. She was a lifelong non-smoker and recalled a single exposure to asbestos when working in a factory 40 years ago. Blood tests demonstrated a persistently raised C-reactive protein (CRP) at 70 mg/dL and otherwise normal parameters including a normal full blood count. A chest X-ray was conducted and is shown in Figure 13.1.

Pleural aspiration under ultrasound (US) guidance was conducted (Figure 13.2) and demonstrated PF protein 38 g/L, glucose 5.7 mmol/L and LDH 191 IU/L. The pleural fluid microbiology was negative, and cytology demonstrated reactive mesothelial cells and some mixed inflammatory cells without a single cell predominance.

a) What is the differential diagnosis?

The presentation post-infectious illness raises the possibility of a reactive effusion or simple/complicated parapneumonic effusion. However, 1 month after treatment and with no lung infiltrate, this is less likely. The pleural fluid biochemical and cytological parameters are against infection with a low lactate dehydrogenase (LDH) and a mixed cell (not neutrophil-dominant) population. Thus, other causes of exudate (including malignancy

DOI: 10.1201/9781003081630-13

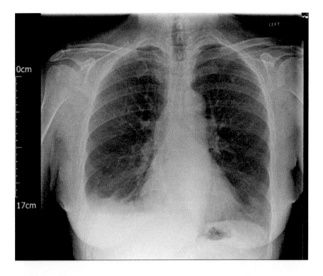

Figure 13.1  Chest X-ray showing a small right pleural effusion.

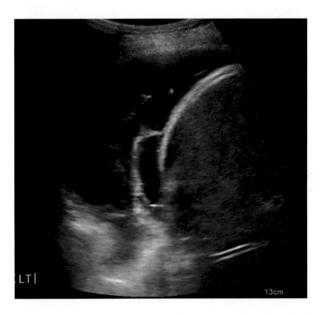

Figure 13.2  US images pre-thoracentesis showing a right pleural effusion with atelectatic lung.

and drug-induced pleural disease given she is on amiodarone) should be considered.

Amiodarone-related effusion usually occurs with lung infiltrates, although isolated effusions have been reported. The pleural fluid in such cases would usually be a lymphocytic exudate (1), although neutrophil-dominant effusions have been reported. Amiodarone-related effusions can be seen late during treatment, but usually occur within 6 years of starting treatment (1,2).

A thoracic CT scan was conducted and is shown in Figure 13.3. The patient underwent local anaesthetic thoracoscopy. At this examination, 800 ml of pleural fluid was drained, and macroscopically there were multiple areas of pleural inflammation and focal pleural lymphangitis, with no evidence of nodularity. Multiple biopsies were taken, and pleural fluid and biopsies were submitted for analysis. The patient was discharged on the same day after full lung expansion.

The pleural fluid and biopsies are shown in Figure 13.4.

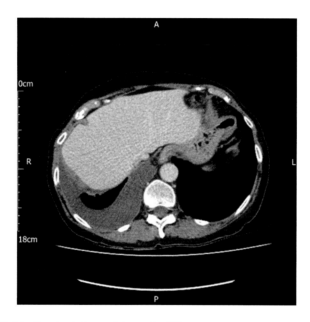

Figure 13.3 Mediastinal view of thoracic CT scan.

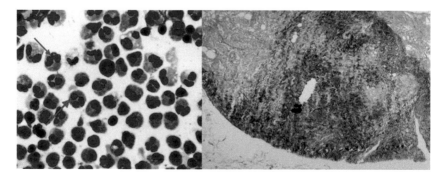

Figure 13.4 (Left) Pleural fluid and (right) pleural biopsy.

b) What do the CT, pleural biopsies and fluid show, and what is the diagnosis?

The CT imaging demonstrates a right basal effusion with some enhancement.

The pleural fluid shows a large number of bilobed nuclei cells consistent with eosinophils (red arrows). The pleural biopsy demonstrates a brisk inflammatory infiltrate.

The diagnosis is consistent with eosinophilic pleuritis.

c) What are the important causes of this condition?

Eosinophilic pleural effusion and pleuritis can be due to several different aetiologies and the differential diagnosis is wide (3,4). The largest case series (of 135 patients from 1,868 patients with pleural effusion) demonstrates that the most common cause of eosinophil pleural effusion is malignancy (seen in 34.8%) and with the majority due to lung carcinoma, followed by infection (19.2% including both parapneumonic effusion and TB), and may be caused by a number of other diseases (autoimmune disease, post-medical or post-surgical procedures, pneumothorax) (5).

A large meta-analysis of the world literature (6) assessed 687 cases of eosinophilic pleural effusion, finding malignancy again as the most common cause (26%) followed by idiopathic (25%) and then parapneumonic (13%). Other causes included blood or air in the pleural space (13%).

The only prospective clinical study in the literature (7) compared eosinophilic effusions to non-eosinophilic effusions (44 and 432 cases, respectively), demonstrating a higher rate of idiopathic disease (25% versus 8%) and post-thoracic surgery (11% versus 3%) in eosinophilic effusions but a similar frequency of malignancy (20.5% and 20.1%).

The cause, in this case, was a likely idiopathic eosinophilic effusion, which we here term 'seronegative eosinophil pleuritis'. It is important to differentiate between a high pleural fluid eosinophil level (>10% of cells in a pleural fluid aspirate) and cases where there is an eosinophilic infiltrate into the parietal pleura (diagnosed only on pleural biopsy). Whereas blood or air in the pleural space is often associated with pleural fluid eosinophils, specific conditions are associated with an eosinophilic parietal pleural infiltrate, and these include idiopathic eosinophilic pleuritis, haematological malignancies and hypereosinophilic syndromes.

In such cases, work-up for autoimmune diseases (including rheumatoid and connective tissue diseases) is important. Drug-induced pleuritis may be considered (and amiodarone was a possible cause in this case, although she had been on this treatment for too long for this to be likely), and in certain situations, parasitic infections should be considered. The well-known conditions of acute and chronic eosinophilic pneumonia only rarely present with significant pleural effusions, although this has been reported (8).

The patient was reviewed with the biopsy results 10 days after the thoracoscopy. Her symptoms initially improved but had returned over a 5-day period. A thoracic ultrasound demonstrated recurrent right pleural fluid.

Further investigations including an autoimmune screen, immunoglobulins and a screen for haematological malignancy were negative. Repeat bloods demonstrated a CRP of 72 mg/dL and a mildly raised peripheral eosinophil count (0.54). A parasite screening was negative.

A diagnosis of idiopathic eosinophilic pleuritis was made. The patient was started on prednisolone treatment (0.5 mg/kg, 30 mg per day) with appropriate counselling for side effects, and treatment for bone and gastric protection was provided.

Two weeks later on treatment, the patient was reviewed again at which point she felt well, with an unlimited exercise tolerance and no systemic symptoms. The CRP had reduced to 10 mg/dL, and the serum eosinophil count was <0.1. Imaging was as shown in Figures 13.5 and 13.6.

d) How do you proceed with treatment?

There are no large-scale studies on eosinophilic pleuritis and steroid treatment. However, in general, these patients require an initial moderate to high dose of steroids (0.5 mg/kg) with appropriate side effect counselling, and other appropriate treatments (gastric and bone protection), followed by a slow wean. In our experience, these patients usually need treatment for about 9 to 12 months, and one should aim for the lowest possible dose of maintenance steroids. Should a significant dose of steroids be required for maintenance, steroid-sparing agents (such as azathioprine) can be considered.

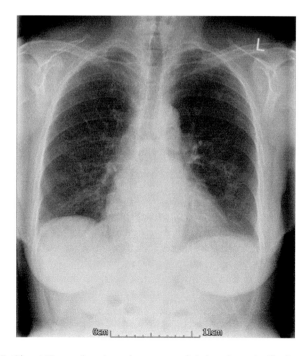

Figure 13.5 Chest X-ray showing clearance of right pleural effusion.

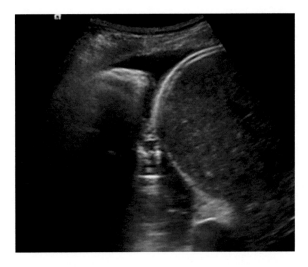

Figure 13.6 Thoracic ultrasound showing small right pleural effusion with underlying lung.

The dose of prednisolone was weaned from 30 mg/day by 5 mg per week and the patient was reviewed on a once-monthly basis. When reviewed at 4 weeks and on 10 mg prednisolone, her symptoms returned and ultrasound demonstrated recurrent pleural fluid.

A slower wean was conducted from 20 mg to 10 mg, weaning by 2 mg per week, but symptoms and fluid returned whenever the steroid dose went below 15 mg/day.

On this basis, the patient was started on azathioprine after Thiopurine Methyltransferase (TMPT) status screening, initially at 1 mg/kg (50 mg) with appropriate liver function and full blood count (FBC) monitoring. After 2 months, the dose was increased to 100 mg, which allowed reduction of the prednisolone dose to 0 mg after 2 months.

The patient remained on azathioprine for a total of 9 months with no evidence of recurrent pleural fluid or symptoms. The azathioprine was eventually stopped 12 months after the initial presentation, with no evidence of recurrent disease after 2 years of further follow-up.

## KEY POINTS

- Eosinophils in pleural fluid have a wide differential diagnosis, including benign conditions but also malignancy.
- Eosinophilic pleuritis, in which case there is an eosinophilic infiltrate into the parietal pleural surface, has a narrower set of differentials including idiopathic, haematological malignancy and autoimmune disease.
- Oral steroid therapy is used in cases of recurrent effusion with an established diagnosis on biopsy and may need to be prolonged.
- Drug-induced pleuritis should be considered in all cases.

# REFERENCES

1. Uong V, Nugent K, Alalawi R, Raj R. Amiodarone-induced loculated pleural effusion: Case report and review of the literature. *Pharmacotherapy* 2010;30(2):218.
2. Carmichael LC, Newman JH. Lymphocytic pleural exudate in a patient receiving amiodarone. *Br J Clin Pract* 1996;50(4):228–30.
3. Kalomenidis I, Light RW. Eosinophilic pleural effusions. *Curr Opin Pulm Med* 2003;9(4):254–60.
4. Kalomenidis I, Light RW. Pathogenesis of the eosinophilic pleural effusions. *Curr Opin Pulm Med* 2004;10(4):289–93.
5. Krenke R, Nasilowski J, Korczynski P, et al. Incidence and aetiology of eosinophilic pleural effusion. *Eur Respir J* 2009;34(5):1111–7.
6. Oba Y, Abu-Salah T. The prevalence and diagnostic significance of eosinophilic pleural effusions: A meta-analysis and systematic review. *Respiration* 2012;83(3):198–208.
7. Rubins JB, Rubins HB. Etiology and prognostic significance of eosinophilic pleural effusions. A prospective study. *Chest* 1996;110(5):1271–4.
8. Samman YS, Wali SO, Abdelaal MA, Gangi MT, Krayem AB. Chronic eosinophilic pneumonia presenting with recurrent massive bilateral pleural effusion: Case report. *Chest* 2001;119(3):968–70.

# 14

# A case of green pleural fluid

RACHELLE ASCIAK

A 79-year-old man, ex-smoker, with a history of hypertension, hypercholester-olaemia and severe peripheral vascular disease, was diagnosed with adenocar-cinoma of the gastro-oesophageal junction. He had been deemed an unsuitable candidate for extensive surgery due to poor performance status and comorbidi-ties, but had undergone palliative radiotherapy for the oesophageal adenocarci-noma 1 year previously and oesophageal stenting 8 months previously. Tumour overgrowth had occurred at the proximal end of the stent causing severe dyspha-gia and a second oesophageal stent was inserted 3 months previously. A com-puted tomography (CT) scan 1 month ago showed a right lower lobe cavitating lung lesion, suspicious for metastatic disease; disease progression with air-fluid level noted at the oesophageal stent; a small area of fluid/air pockets around the stent; and a large right-sided pleural effusion.

He was referred to respiratory in view of the large, unilateral, right-sided pleu-ral effusion (Figure 14.1). The main symptom at the time was acid reflux causing intermittent cough. A bedside thoracic ultrasound demonstrated a large, right-sided pleural effusion, five rib spaces deep, with 15 cm maximum depth, mod-erately echogenic and with no septations. A total of 1000 ml of greenish fluid (Figure 14.2) was drained, after which the patient developed chest discomfort, which led to terminating the fluid drainage procedure.

a) What is the differential diagnosis?

The most likely differential diagnoses of a large unilateral pleural effu-sion in a patient with underlying progressive malignancy are a malignant pleural effusion, pleural infection and chylothorax. However, the patient did not have any infective symptoms, the fluid was odourless and the colour of the fluid was not the typical white/cream appearance of a chylothorax. The colour of the pleural fluid drained raised suspicion of possible biliothorax.

DOI: 10.1201/9781003081630-14

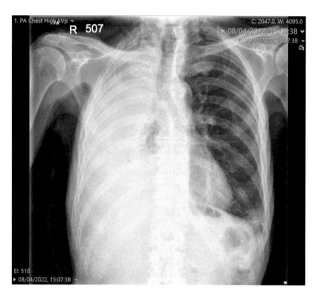

Figure 14.1  Chest X-ray showing a large, right-sided pleural effusion.

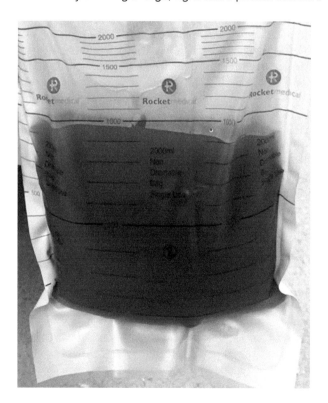

Figure 14.2  The green-coloured pleural fluid drained.

b) What is biliothorax?

Biliothorax (also referred to as cholethorax, pleurobilia and thoracobilia in the literature) is the accumulation of bile within the pleural cavity. It is uncommon with about 60 reported cases in the literature (1). It is most commonly reported as a consequence of bile duct injury or subphrenic abscess formation, and causes include blunt and penetrating diaphragmatic trauma, complication of percutaneous hepatobiliary drain insertion, complication of hepatobiliary malignancy, and parasitic infections such as hepatic hydatidosis and amoebiasis (1–5).

Biliothorax more commonly occurs on the right. Bile is alkaline and therefore caustic to the pleura. Echinococcus cysts produce proteolytic enzymes, and subsequent corrosion of the diaphragm may explain some cases of biliothorax which do not have evidence of iatrogenic or traumatic perforating injury (1, 6).

c) What further investigations can help confirm the suspected diagnosis?

The suspicion of biliothorax can be confirmed by a pleural fluid-to-serum bilirubin ratio of >1. Other investigations may include a CT scan, which may identify a fistula; and magnetic resonance cholangiopancreatography (MRCP) and endoscopic retrograde cholangiopancreatography (ERCP), which may reveal contrast spillage from the biliary tree into the pleural cavity and can confirm the diagnosis, with ERCP also allowing the insertion of stents/stone removal/sphincterotomy if required. Surgery may be both diagnostic and therapeutic, allowing the repair of defects found during surgery (2, 7–9).

d) What is the best way of managing biliothorax?

A biliothorax should be drained due to the risk of development of empyema, non-expandable lung or acute respiratory distress syndrome (ARDS), as bile irritates the lung and pleura. In addition, consideration should be given to fluid and nutritional support and antibiotic cover. Further management is dictated according to the underlying cause.

In this case, the patient was too frail for further investigation, and he died soon after of progressive malignant disease. The presumed mechanism for biliothorax was either through the right lower lobe cavitating lung metastasis, having eroded through the diaphragm and caused a biliopleural fistula, or possible erosion of tumour/oesophageal stent into the pleura, and bile reflux in the stomach and oesophagus, spilling over into the pleura at the level of the stent.

## KEY POINTS

- Biliothorax is rare and occurs when bile accumulates within the pleural cavity, most commonly after trauma or as a complication of hepatobiliary malignancy or surgery, or parasitic infections.
- Biliothorax presents as a unilateral, most commonly right-sided, pleural effusion, and the pleural fluid has a green tint. The pleural fluid-to-serum bilirubin ratio is >1.

- Biliothorax is associated with risk of empyema and should be drained. Further treatment should be directed at the underlying cause and may include gastroenterology and surgical interventions, with close liaison with other services.

## REFERENCES

1. Adam A, Fox N, Terrill Huggins J, Chopra A. The Green Pleural Effusion: A Comprehensive Review of the Bilothorax with Case Series. *PLEURA*. 2017 December;4:21–31.
2. Asad Ali K, Abid J. Bilio-Thorax: An Unrecognised Complication of Liver Surgery. *Int J Surg Case Rep*. 2020 May 14;71:346–8.
3. Sano A, Yotsumoto T. Bilothorax as a Complication of Percutaneous Transhepatic Biliary Drainage. *Asian Cardiovasc Thorac Ann*. 2016 January;24(1):101–3.
4. Ibarra-Pérez C. Thoracic Complications of Amebic Abscess of the Liver: Report of 501 Cases. *Chest*. 1981 June 1;79(6):672–7.
5. Kabiri EH, El Maslout A, Benosman A. Thoracic Rupture of Hepatic Hydatidosis (123 Cases). *Ann Thorac Surg*. 2001 December;72(6):1883–6.
6. Kolbakir F, Erk MK, Keçeligil HT, Yilman M. Cholethorax. *J Exp Clin Med*. 2009 December 22;11(1): 45–6.
7. Ragozzino A, De Rosa R, Galdiero R, Maio A, Manes G. Bronchobiliary Fistula Evaluated with Magnetic Resonance Imaging. *Acta Radiol*. 2005 January 1;46(5):452–4.
8. Karabulut N, Çakmak V, Kiter G. Confident Diagnosis of Bronchobiliary Fistula Using Contrast-Enhanced Magnetic Resonance Cholangiography. *Korean J Radiol*. 2010;11(4):493–6.
9. Soler-Sempere MJ. An Unusual Case of Left-Sided Massive Biliothorax. *Int J Respir Pulm Med*. 2015 December;2(4).

# 15

# Pleural effusion in a patient with previous pancreatitis

## VINEETH GEORGE

A 76-year-old gentleman was referred to the respiratory service with a 2-month history of progressive breathlessness. He was diagnosed with IgG4-related auto-immune pancreatitis at the age of 70 after histology from a Whipple's resection demonstrated lymphoplasmacytic sclerosing pancreatitis with an elevated serum IgG4 level. Immunohistochemistry at the time revealed CD3-positive T cells along with clusters of IgG4-positive plasma cells (120 per high power field in hot spots). He was a retired electrician with a known history of occupational asbestos exposure. He had not experienced any systemic symptoms such as weight loss or fevers and had no known contact with tuberculosis.

A recent CT chest demonstrated parietal pleural thickening bilaterally with left pleural effusion and mediastinal adenopathy (Figure 15.1). He subsequently underwent a thoracocentesis and an ultrasound-guided biopsy of the left pleura.

a) What are the features of pulmonary and pleural IgG4 and how is it diagnosed?

IgG4-related disease (IgG4-RD) is a fibroinflammatory condition that was first described as a distinct disease in the last 20 years (1). It was first described in the pancreas (1, 2), and patients typically present with gastrointestinal symptoms (3). However, it can affect virtually any organ including the lungs, pleura and mediastinum. IgG4-RD can be localised to individual organs or present with systemic disease (4).

It is predominantly seen in men, with a median age of 60–65 years (4). Patients with IgG4-RD typically present with symptoms related to the organs involved, which can include the pancreas, bile ducts, lacrimal glands, salivary gland, thyroid, lung, liver and kidney, or with abnormal imaging or laboratory findings.

DOI: 10.1201/9781003081630-15

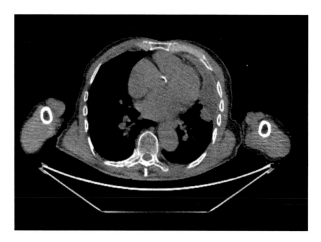

Figure 15.1 Mediastinal window of thoracic CT.

Retrospective cohort data suggest that thoracic involvement is seen in approximately half of all patients with IgG4-RD (5). Although the precise degree of pleural involvement is unknown, data from small cohorts have suggested that this can be as high as 16% (3, 5).

Small series of patients with pleural effusions that were undiagnosed during long-term follow-up have demonstrated elevated IgG4 levels in the effusion with marked plasma cell infiltration in the pleura (6, 7). The largest of these series found that 36% met the diagnostic criteria for IgG4-RD (6).

Elevated serum IgG4 levels were considered to be the hallmark of the disease but may not be elevated in half of all individuals with biologically active, biopsy-proven disease (8). Elevated serum IgG4 levels may also be seen in 5% of all normal individuals (8). Cohort data from the UK suggest that higher serum IgG4 levels were associated with thoracic disease, possibly providing evidence of greater disease activity (3). Similarly, data from small case series suggest that inflammatory markers such as C-reactive protein and lactate dehydrogenase (LDH) are either normal or only modestly elevated (9). Effusions are typically lymphocytic and high pleural fluid adenosine deaminase (ADA) levels have been reported (9).

Imaging features of thoracic involvement in IgG4-RD are often non-specific. Hilar and mediastinal lymphadenopathy are the most common manifestations and are seen in approximately half of all cases and in the majority of patients with thoracic involvement (3, 5). Cohort data suggest that lung nodules and bronchovascular manifestations are seen in approximately a quarter of patients, with pleural manifestations affecting up to 16% (5). These can include pleural effusion, pleural thickening and pleural-based masses (5, 9). IgG4-RD pericarditis is considered rarer, with data largely limited to case reports and small series (5, 10).

Pleural effusions in IgG4-RD are exudates which are rich in lymphocytes (11). However, the differential for IgG4-RD is broad and includes a number of fibro-inflammatory multi-system disorders such as sarcoidosis, connective tissue disease, Castleman's disease, and both solid organ tumours and lymphoma (3). Biopsies have traditionally been recommended in consensus guidelines to exclude malignancies and other inflammatory processes (12–14).

The characteristic histological features of IgG4-RD are a dense lympho-plasmocytic infiltrate, obliterative phlebitis and storiform fibrosis. Plasma cell infiltration with >10 IgG4-positive plasma cells/high power field and an IgG4/IgG-positive plasma cell ratio of more than 40% are suggestive of IgG4-RD for biopsied specimens (12). Features such as a prominent neutrophilic infiltrate, abscess, necrosis and epithelioid cell granuloma are less consistent with a diagnosis of IgG4-RD (6).

However, it should be noted that current guidelines from the American League of Rheumatology and the European League Against Rheumatism do not require a biopsy to diagnose IgG4-RD in patients thought to have 'straightforward' clinical, radiological and serological findings (15). Furthermore, 37% of patients classified with IgG4 under the American and European classification lacked the classical histopathological findings and more than 40% did not meet previously determined cut-offs for IgG4-positive plasma cell infiltrates (15).

The pleural fluid chemistry was exudative with no malignant cells seen on cytology. Pleural biopsy demonstrated fibrotic pleura and patchy minor acute and chronic inflammation. There was no evidence of malignancy and granulomas were not seen. There was no storiform fibrosis or obliterative phlebitis. A very scanty lymphoplasmacytic infiltrate with IgG4 immunostaining revealed a maximum of eight positive plasma cells per high power field, and an IgG4:IgG ratio of 30% was reported. The biopsy was thought to have no specific features suggestive of IgG4-RD.

He remained under imaging surveillance for approximately 1 year but subsequently developed a large circumferential pericardial effusion. He underwent pericardiocentesis and was found to have exudative changes within the pericardium and was treated with colchicine with good clinical response.

He remains under the care of a subspecialist IgG4 clinic with annual monitoring of his serum IgG4 levels and serial PET scans to ascertain disease activity.

This case highlights the diagnostic challenges associated with this condition. Although he has evidence of multi-site serositis, radiology consistent with thoracic IgG4-RD and a history of known pancreatic IgG4-RD, his pleural biopsy results are atypical for IgG4-RD. Consequently, the diagnosis for his pleural disease is unclear and this may be viewed differently depending on which guideline or consensus classification is applied.

b) How do you treat IgG4-RD?

There is limited high-quality data to guide treatment approaches and most of the existing literature is based on small East Asian studies. Isolated pleural involvement is thought to typically follow a benign course (11). Some patients may show spontaneous remission, however, consensus guidelines recommend that those with other organ involvement should be offered treatment due to the risk of progression to irreversible end-organ dysfunction (13).

Corticosteroids are considered first-line treatment and Japanese guidelines recommend commencing patients on 0.5–0.6mg/kg per day with a gradual taper depending on clinical and radiological response. A small Chinese randomised controlled trial comparing doses of 0.5–0.6 mg/kg to 0.8–1.0 mg/kg found no difference in rates of relapse, although this trial was limited by a small sample size, with 20 participants in each arm, and an open-label design (16). A high relapse rate is seen with this therapy and a maintenance dose of 5–10mg has been recommended (17). Although a clear alternative to corticosteroids has not been established, rituximab, a beta cell-depleting monoclonal, has been found to produce disease responses in retrospective and open-label trials (18, 19).

## KEY POINTS

- IgG4-RD is a recently described multi-system fibroinflammatory disorder which can affect the pleura.
- Diagnosis can be challenging and typically involves clinical, radiological, serological and pathological domains.
- There is minimal data to guide treatment strategies, but corticosteroids are considered first-line.

## REFERENCES

1. Yoshida K, Toki F, Takeuchi T, Watanabe SI, Shiratori K, Hayashi N. Chronic pancreatitis caused by an autoimmune abnormality. Proposal of the concept of autoimmune pancreatitis. *Dig Dis Sci.* 1995 July;40(7):1561–8.
2. Hamano H, Kawa S, Horiuchi A, et al. High serum IgG4 concentrations in patients with sclerosing pancreatitis. *N Engl J Med.* 2001;344(10):732–738.
3. Corcoran JP, Culver EL, Anstey RM, Talwar A, Manganis CD, Cargill TN, et al. Thoracic involvement in IgG4-related disease in a UK-based patient cohort. *Respir Med.* 2017 November 1;132:117–21.
4. Ryu JH, Sekiguchi H, Yi ES. Pulmonary manifestations of immunoglobulin G4-related sclerosing disease. *Eur Respir J.* 2012;39(1):180–6.

5. Fei Y, Shi J, Lin W, Chen Y, Feng R, Wu Q, et al. Intrathoracic involvements of immunoglobulin G4-related sclerosing disease. *Medicine (United States)*. 2015;94(50):e2150.
6. Murata Y, Aoe K, Mimura-Kimura Y, Murakami T, Oishi K, Matsumoto T, et al. Association of immunoglobulin G4 and free light chain with idiopathic pleural effusion. *Clin Exp Immunol*. 2017 October 1;190(1):133–42.
7. Kasashima S, Kawashima A, Ozaki S, Kita T, Araya T, Ohta Y, et al. Clinicopathological features of immunoglobulin G4-related pleural lesions and diagnostic utility of pleural effusion cytology. *Cytopathology*. 2019 May 8;30(3):285–94.
8. Wallace ZS, Deshpande V, Mattoo H, Mahajan VS, Kulikova M, Pillai S, et al. IgG4-related disease: Clinical and laboratory features in one hundred twenty-five patients. *Arthritis Rheumatol*. 2015 September 1;67(9):2466–75.
9. Saito Z, Yoshida M, Kojima A, Tamura K, Kuwano K. Characteristics of pleural effusion in IgG4-related pleuritis. *Respir Med Case Rep*. 2020 January 1;29: 101019.
10. Doumen M, Vankelecom B, Westhovens R, Michiels S. Pericarditis as a manifestation of IgG4-related disease. *Rheumatol Int*. 2022;42(7):1287–95.
11. Murata Y, Aoe K, Mimura Y. Pleural effusion related to IgG4. *Curr Opin Pulm Med*. 2019;25(4):384–90.
12. Deshpande V, Zen Y, Chan JKC, Yi EE, Sato Y, Yoshino T, et al. Consensus statement on the pathology of IgG4-related disease. *Mod Pathol*. 2012 September;25(9):1181–92.
13. Khosroshahi A, Wallace ZS, Crowe JL, Akamizu T, Azumi A, Carruthers MN, et al. International consensus guidance statement on the management and treatment of IgG4-related disease. *Arthritis Rheumatol*. 2015 July;67(7):1688–99.
14. Umehara H, Okazaki K, Kawa S, Takahashi H, Goto H, Matsui S, et al. The 2020 revised comprehensive diagnostic (RCD) criteria for IgG4-RD. *Mod Rheumatol*. 2021;31(3):529–33.
15. Wallace ZS, Naden RP, Chari S, Choi H, Della-Torre E, Dicaire JF, et al. The 2019 American College of Rheumatology/European League Against Rheumatism classification criteria for IgG4-related disease. *Arthritis Rheumatol*. 2020 January 1;72(1):7–19.
16. Wu Q, Chang J, Chen H, Chen Y, Yang H, Fei Y, et al. Efficacy between high and medium doses of glucocorticoid therapy in remission induction of IgG4-related diseases: A preliminary randomized controlled trial. *Int J Rheum Dis*. 2017 May 1;20(5):639–46.
17. Masaki Y, Shimizu H, Nakamura TS, Nakamura T, Nakajima A, Kawanami HI, et al. IgG4-related disease: Diagnostic methods and therapeutic strategies in Japan. *J Clin Exp Hematop*. 2014;54(2): 95–101.

18. Ebbo M, Grados A, Samson M, Groh M, Loundou A, Rigolet A, et al. Long-term efficacy and safety of rituximab in IgG4-related disease: Data from a French nationwide study of thirty-three patients. *PLOS ONE*. 2017 September 15;12(9):e0183844.
19. Carruthers MN, Topazian MD, Khosroshahi A, Witzig TE, Wallace ZS, Hart PA, et al. Rituximab for IgG4-related disease: A prospective, open-label trial. *Ann Rheum Dis*. 2015 June;74(6):1171–7.

# 16

# Pleural effusion and abnormal bones

NAJIB M RAHMAN

A 44-year-old woman presented with right-sided pleuritic chest pain on the background of right-sided shoulder pain. She had received 5 days of antibiotics from the GP with no improvement. There was no other medical history other than a 2-year history of right-sided shoulder pain which had been slowly progressive and treated with analgesia.

a) What does the chest X-ray show (Figure 16.1)?

The chest X-ray demonstrates a large right pleural effusion, but volume loss in addition in the right apex, and absence of the second to the fifth ribs.

A right-sided pleural effusion was confirmed on ultrasound (US), a large volume aspiration (1600 ml) was performed with US guidance (Figure 16.2) and a thoracic CT scan was performed. Baseline blood parameters, including inflammatory markers, were normal.

The thoracic US demonstrated an echogenic effusion with no pleural thickening and normal diaphragm function. The pleural aspiration fluid demonstrated straw-coloured fluid which was an exudate (PF protein 43 g/L, glucose 5.4 mmol/L, LDH 134 IU/L) with normal triglyceride levels (0.3 mmol/L). Pleural fluid microbiology was negative, and cytology demonstrated a mixed inflammatory cell population with small lymphocytes and occasional neutrophils and eosinophils.

The thoracic CT demonstrated normal lung parenchyma, and no evidence of pleural enhancement or thickening (Figure 16.3).

b) What is the differential diagnosis at this stage and what is your next diagnostic step?

The differential diagnosis for the pleural effusion remains wide at this stage, with the presence of a non-inflammatory exudate in an otherwise fit and

DOI: 10.1201/9781003081630-16

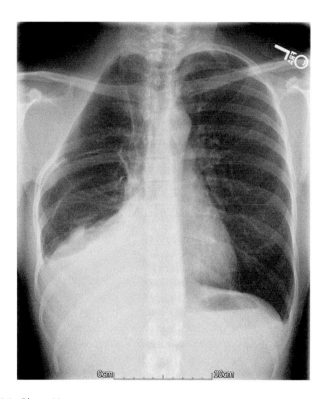

Figure 16.1 Chest X-ray.

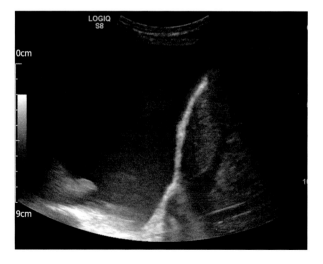

Figure 16.2 Right-sided thoracic ultrasound image.

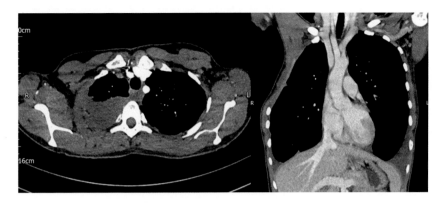

Figure 16.3 CT showing a mediastinal and coronal view of the thorax.

well young woman. The clinical presentation and normal fluid LDH (lactate dehydrogenase) make infection unlikely, the biochemical parameters do not suggest pleural TB, and malignancy, inflammatory disease and other causes remain on the differential diagnosis. Chylothorax has been effectively excluded by both the macroscopic appearance of the fluid (although a minority of chylothorax can be associated with normal macroscopic appearances) and the fluid triglyceride level. Autoimmune disease should be considered, but the patient does not report pleuritic symptoms and hence conditions such as systemic lupus erythematosus (SLE) are less likely (whereas rheumatoid pleuritis which is typically painless remains on the differential diagnosis).

The CT also demonstrates a small left effusion and absence of the second to fifth ribs. Malignant disease would not cause this appearance of complete absence of the ribs, and the differential includes congenital absence of the ribs (normal variant, Down's syndrome, Poland syndrome) but this usually does not affect so many ribs, or a rib destructive condition.

Given an undiagnosed exudate with a non-informative CT scan, pleural biopsy and further bone imaging should be the next diagnostic step.

The patient underwent a local anaesthetic thoracoscopy which demonstrated mild pleural inflammation only with no nodularity or thickening (Figure 16.4). Multiple pleural biopsies demonstrated mild fibrosis and a chronic inflammatory cell infiltrate.

An MRI of the spine and thorax was conducted (Figure 16.5).

c) What is now the most likely diagnosis and how is this confirmed?

The MRI spine demonstrates diffuse high T1 signal change between C3 and C7 (blue arrow), and other images (not displayed) showed complete osteolysis of the right second to fourth ribs. The presence of bone destruction (as opposed to congenital absence) and pleural effusion raises the possibility of Gorham–Stout disease (GSD), also known as vanishing bone disease.

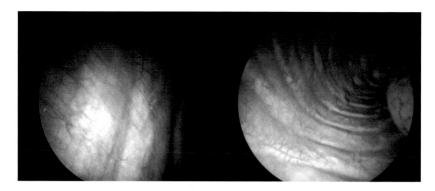

Figure 16.4 Thoracoscopic view of the pleural surface.

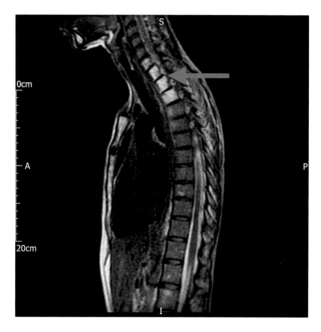

Figure 16.5 Sagittal view of MRI cervicothoracic spine.

There is no single diagnostic test for GSD, but the diagnosis is supported by a biopsy demonstrating non-malignant hyperproliferation of blood vessels (1).

Based on the aforementioned information, the patient underwent a CT-guided biopsy of the lytic portion of the C7 vertebra. The biopsies demonstrated minimal included bone which was D2-40 staining positive, and there was evidence of vascular proliferation.

Despite the biopsy being non-supportive, a diagnosis of thoracic GSD was made.

d) What is the cause of this condition and what is the treatment?

GSD is a rare idiopathic disease which causes progressive osteolysis, and benign lymphatic, fibrotic and vascular tissue proliferation (2), potentially related to increased cytokines such as IL-6, first reported in a case series in 1955 (3). GSD usually presents in adolescence but can present at any age and is associated with chylothorax in up to 20% of cases, thought secondary to disease invasion of the thoracic duct adjacent to the spine. Typical biopsy findings include lymphatic and vascular tissue within bone (4) and positive staining for D2-40 (a lymphatic endothelial marker) on immunohistochemistry. Spine and thoracic involvement together is rare (5).

Treatment is supportive, with drainage of the fluid according to symptoms (and some authorities using pleurodesis) and then suppression of osteoclast activity. This is usually conducted with a combination of bisphosphonates and vitamin D, with radiotherapy sometimes considered for bony lesions. As there is some evidence of abnormality of the mTOR pathway, mTOR inhibitors have been used (6,7).

Due to the multi-site lesions (rib, spine), radiotherapy was not an option. The patient went on to be treated with monthly zoledronic acid infusions, and started treatment with sirolimus, increasing in dose from 2 mg initially to 6 mg per day to achieve a serum drug level of 8–15 ng/mL.

e) What particular complications should be looked for in this case?

Symptoms including breathlessness should be screened for and the pleural fluid drained as required. The absence of the ribs with associated volume loss in the right hemithorax requires consideration – this could potentially lead to respiratory and ventilatory failure, and regular screening for sleep-related symptoms (such as nocturnal hypoventilation) should be conducted.

The patient was treated as noted and is stable 2 years after diagnosis on a regime of monthly bisphosphonates and sirolimus. Repeat ultrasound demonstrated complete resolution of the right effusion, with a modest amount of benign-looking pleural thickening. Repeat MRI imaging demonstrated no progression of the signal intensity in the vertebra and no further bone destruction.

## KEY POINTS

- GSD is a rare clinical entity, but a known cause of pleural effusion, specifically of chylothorax.
- The diagnosis should be suspected in an undiagnosed exudate in the presence of bone abnormalities either concurrently or in the previous history.

- Treatment involves liaison with local or regional specialists in metabolic bone disease, mechanical drainage of pleural fluid and sometimes use of mTOR inhibitors.

## REFERENCES

1. Nikolaou VS, Chytas D, Korres D, Efstathopoulos N. Vanishing bone disease (Gorham-Stout syndrome): A review of a rare entity. *World J Orthop* 2014;5(5):694–698.
2. Wang P, Liao W, Cao G, Jiang Y. A rare case of Gorham-Stout syndrome involving the thoracic spine with progressive bilateral chylothorax: A case report. *BMC Musculoskelet Disord* 2019;20(1):154.
3. Gorham LW, Stout AP. Massive osteolysis (acute spontaneous absorption of bone, phantom bone, disappearing bone); its relation to hemangiomatosis. *J Bone Joint Surg Am* 1955;37-A(5):985–1004.
4. Dellinger MT, Garg N, Olsen BR. Viewpoints on vessels and vanishing bones in Gorham-Stout disease. *Bone* 2014;63:47–52.
5. Koto K, Inui K, Itoi M, Itoh K. Gorham-Stout disease in the rib and thoracic spine with spinal injury treated with radiotherapy, zoledronic acid, vitamin D, and propranolol: A case report and literature review. *Mol Clin Oncol* 2019;11(6):551–556.
6. Hagendoorn J, Yock TI, Borel Rinkes IH, Padera TP, Ebb DH. Novel molecular pathways in Gorham disease: Implications for treatment. *Pediatr Blood Cancer* 2014;61(3):401–406.
7. Liang Y, Tian R, Wang J, et al. Gorham-Stout disease successfully treated with sirolimus (rapamycin): A case report and review of the literature. *BMC Musculoskelet Disord* 2020;21(1):577.

# 17

# Pleural effusion in a patient with chronic myeloid leukaemia

DINESH ADDALA

A 68-year-old woman presented to the pleural service with breathlessness and an exercise tolerance of less than 100 metres, progressive over 3 weeks. She complained of an occasional dry cough but no fevers, chest pain or loss of appetite/weight.

Her past medical history included chronic myeloid leukaemia (CML) and seronegative inflammatory arthritis, but an otherwise performance status of 1. Her medications included dasatinib and hydroxychloroquine, both of which she had been on for over 5 years.

Thoracic ultrasound of the right side is illustrated in Figure 17.1.

a) Describe the ultrasound findings and explain why this patient is breathless.

The ultrasound illustrates a large, right-sided pleural effusion, with an atelectatic lung (blue star) and flattened hemidiaphragm (blue arrow). As this ultrasound was taken during thoracocentesis, the pleural aspiration catheter is also visible (white arrow).

The patient is likely to be breathless due to flattening of the diaphragm, which is demonstrated on ultrasound imaging. The Pleural Effusion and Symptom Evaluation (PLEASE) study found that breathlessness relief post-aspiration was independently associated with baseline abnormal/paralyzed/paradoxical diaphragm movement (odds ratio 4.37) (1).

She underwent pleural aspiration and subsequent CT scan (Figure 17.2) and the results are as follows:

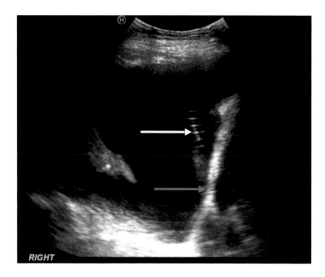

Figure 17.1 Right-sided thoracic ultrasound.

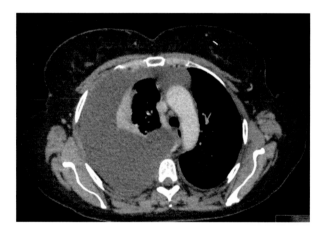

Figure 17.2 CT scan, mediastinal window.

Pleural fluid protein 47 g/L, glucose 5.8 mmol/L, LDH 171 IU/L.

*Cytology*: small lymphocytes without atypia. In the MGG-stained (May Grunwald-Giemsa) section, there are moderate amounts of blood. A few clusters of mildly atypical epithelioid cells are seen, interpreted as reactive mesothelial cells given the inflammation. No obviously malignant cells are seen.

b) What are the key findings and what are the possible differential diagnoses?

The CT scan shows a large, unilateral, right-sided pleural effusion with no discernible pleural nodularity or thickening. There are no other obvious mass lesions.

The pleural fluid is exudative without overt biochemical evidence of infection (normal glucose and low/normal lactate dehydrogenase [LDH]). The cytology does not demonstrate malignant cells.

The differential diagnosis is wide here, with possibilities including pleural effusion related to the patient's known CML, related to inflammatory arthritis (inflammatory) or medication. A new malignancy should also be considered.

c) What is the evidence-based strategy to proceed with the investigation and management of this patient?

Recent evidence has shown the overall sensitivity of pleural fluid cytology to be low, in particular with cancers such as mesothelioma (<5%) (2,3). As such, the presence of a cytology negative exudative pleural effusion should prompt consideration of a biopsy. In this case, the patient is of good performance status, and the highest yield would be via local anaesthetic (medical) thoracoscopy or surgical thoracoscopy, with a diagnostic yield of approximately 95% (4).

Thoracoscopy demonstrated inflammatory appearances, with parietal pleural thickening in areas but no nodularity or malignant changes. Histology of pleural biopsies demonstrated fibrosis and inflammation with no granulomas or malignancy. The pleural effusion was recurrent despite drainage of 1,500 ml at thoracoscopy.

d) What is the most likely diagnosis and what are the next steps?

The most likely diagnosis is a dasatinib-related pleural effusion. Dasatinib is a tyrosine kinase inhibitor (TKI) used in the treatment of CML. The DASISION (Dasatinib versus Imatinib Study in Treatment-Naïve CML Patients) (5) found that 28% of patients treated with dasatinib developed pleural effusion of any grade (5-year follow-up) with similar results from the CA180-034 study (6) (7-year follow-up) with 33% developing pleural effusion. The pleural effusion rate with the tyrosine kinase inhibitor imatinib is 1%, suggesting a specific drug effect rather than a wider class effect.

It is important to note that a long history of dasatinib treatment does not rule out dasatinib-related pleural effusion, with the aforementioned studies finding the median time to drug-related pleural effusion being 114 weeks in DASISION and 60 weeks in CA180-034.

The next step in management is to closely monitor the patient after a trial of stopping or dose-reducing dasatinib to assess the impact on pleural effusion (and CML progression) in liaison with the haematology team.

The patient was reviewed by the pleural service 2 months later and was found to have only a small basal pleural effusion, with no respiratory symptoms. A contemporaneous haematology review found the BCR-ABL gene level to have increased significantly.

e) What should be the next step in treatment?

The patient has responded well to cessation of dasatinib treatment in terms of pleural effusion, however, the consequence is that the CML status has deteriorated. She requires further TKI treatment, and the options include introduction of an alternative TKI such as imatinib or cautiously restarting dasatinib at a lower dose.

As the patient had previously suffered intolerable side effects with imatinib, the decision was made to commence dasatinib at a dose of 50 mg daily (50% dose reduction) and monitor the clinical situation.

Over the next 2 years, the patient was largely stable. Attempts to up-titrate the dasatinib to 100 mg daily were unsuccessful with recurrence of pleural effusion; she continued on 50 mg per day thereafter.

She re-presented acutely to hospital 2 years later with a new left (contralateral)-sided pleural effusion. This was drained and once again found to be a cytology negative exudate. Given the known history of dasatinib-related pleural effusion, rather than undertake thoracoscopy, the decision was made to hold dasatinib as a trial and assess pleural effusion size. Once again, the pleural effusion resolved with dasatinib cessation, and a subsequent trial of half-dose treatment failed with repeated pleural effusion requiring drainage.

Given the requirement for treatment with TKI for her CML, it was thus necessary to switch her to bosutinib, which was successful with good disease control and no pleural effusion recurrence.

Dasatinib-induced pleural effusion is an important cause of pleural effusion and should be considered in all patients on the drug presenting with new pleural effusion. Treating clinicians should be aware that pleural effusion can present at any time during the treatment course of dasatinib, even years after commencement. Few formal guidelines exist; close collaboration between haematologists and respiratory physicians is required both in the investigation pathway and management (7). Note the following management principles:

1) A careful clinical history and examination.
2) Investigation of a unilateral pleural effusion that does not resolve with dasatinib cessation.
3) Small or asymptomatic dasatinib-related effusions, once the diagnosis is secured and other pleural causes excluded, can be monitored 3–6 monthly with chest radiographs and thoracic ultrasound. Dose reduction may be considered if symptoms develop and CML response remains adequate on the lower dose.
4) For moderate or large pleural effusions, interrupting treatment to assess response in pleural effusion, then restarting at a lower dose (e.g. 50 mg/day) is reasonable, and some patients may tolerate up-titration to full dose again. CML disease control should be actively monitored.
5) If lower doses of dasatinib are not tolerated with the need for recurrent pleural aspirations (typically more than two), consider switching treatment to an alternative TKI in discussion with the haematology team.

## KEY POINTS

- Symptoms of pleural effusion are particularly significant in the presence of a flattened or paradoxically moving diaphragm.
- The differential diagnosis of pleural effusion in the presence of haematological malignancy is wide, but drug-related effusion should be considered.
- After the exclusion of other causes (including by biopsy), dasatinib-related pleural effusion is a common cause of effusion in CML patients.
- Treatment includes cessation of the drug and may require restart at lower doses.

## REFERENCES

1. Muruganandan S, Azzopardi M, Thomas R, et al. The Pleural Effusion And Symptom Evaluation (PLEASE) study of breathlessness in patients with a symptomatic pleural effusion. *Eur Respir J* 2020;55(5):1900980.
2. Arnold DT, De Fonseka D, Perry S, et al. Investigating unilateral pleural effusions: The role of cytology. *Eur Respir J* 2018;52(5):1801254.
3. Mercer R, Varatharajah R, Shepherd G, et al. Critical analysis of the utility of initial pleural aspiration in the diagnosis and management of suspected malignant pleural effusion. *BMJ Open Respir Res* 2020;7(1):e000701.
4. Hooper C, Lee GYC, Maskell NA, BTS Pleural Guideline Group. Investigation of a unilateral pleural effusion in adults: British Thoracic Society pleural disease guideline 2010. In: BTS pleural disease guideline. *Thorax* 2010;65 Supplement 2:ii4–ii17.
5. Cortes JE, Saglio G, Kantarjian HM, et al. Final 5-year study results of DASISION: The Dasatinib versus Imatinib Study in Treatment-Naïve Chronic Myeloid Leukemia Patients trial. *J Clin Oncol* 2016;34(20):2333–2340.
6. Shah NP, Rousselot P, Schiffer C, et al. Dasatinib in Imatinib-resistant or -intolerant chronic-phase, chronic myeloid leukemia patients: 7-year follow-up of study CA180-034. *Am J Hematol* 2016;91(9):869–874.
7. Cortes JE, Jimenez CA, Mauro MJ, Geyer A, Pinilla-Ibarz J, Smith BD. Pleural effusion in dasatinib-treated patients with chronic myeloid leukemia in chronic phase: Identification and management. *Clin Lymphoma Myeloma Leuk* 2017;17(2):78–82.

# 18

# An unusual pleural abnormality

RACHELLE ASCIAK

An 80-year-old man, non-smoker, with a history of hypertension presented with a 1-month history of intermittent vague left-sided chest pains, not related to exertion or to the time of day. He had noticed some shortness of breath on strenuous exertion during the previous year but otherwise felt relatively well. He recalled having been exposed to asbestos in the past when working in a dockyard.

A chest X-ray requested to investigate the chest pain showed left-sided blunting of the costophrenic angle in keeping with a small left-sided pleural effusion and he was therefore referred to pleural clinic. When reviewed, a thoracic ultrasound was performed and this identified a small, non-echogenic, left-sided effusion with 3 cm maximum depth and seen in only one rib space. A 2 cm diameter, well-circumscribed, hypodense round pleural lesion (Figures 18.1 and 18.2) was identified. A thoracic CT scan demonstrated small volume pleural plaques, a small left-sided pleural effusion and a posterior pleural nodule arising from the parietal pleura (Figure 18.3), without chest wall invasion and without pleural thickening over the mediastinal pleural surface. No other abnormalities were seen on the CT scan.

a) What is the differential diagnosis?

The differential diagnosis of a solitary pleural nodule includes metastasis from a primary malignancy elsewhere, localised malignant mesothelioma, sarcoma, pleural lymphoma, peripheral lung nodule/neoplasm, solitary fibrous tumour of the pleura (SFTP), splenosis, lipoma and mesothelial cyst (1). Occasionally, localised pleural thickening or pleural plaque may appear as a solitary pleural nodule.

Solitary fibrous tumours of the pleura are rare, account for <5% of pleural tumours and usually arise from the visceral pleura (1, 2). They usually appear

DOI: 10.1201/9781003081630-18

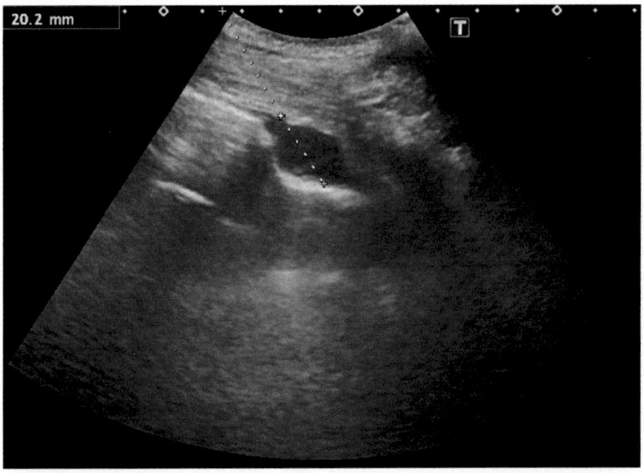

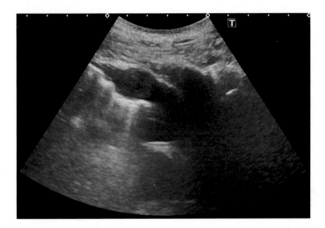

Figure 18.1 Ultrasound image of the well-circumscribed, 2 cm in diameter, rounded pleural lesion.

Figure 18.2 Ultrasound image of the well-circumscribed, 2 cm in diameter, rounded pleural lesion.

as well-demarcated peripheral lesions abutting the pleura with a broad base or, more commonly, a pedicle, and forming an obtuse angle with the pleural surface (3). Malignant histological features are found in 30%, with most SFTP considered benign, however, in a systematic review including 1,542 SFTP, 2.8% of patients with resected 'benign' histology SFTP experienced recurrence (2).

b) What is the optimal investigation of a solitary pleural nodule?

Investigation plans depend on the associated clinical and radiological features. A PET CT scan may be able to differentiate benign from malignant causes, and a biopsy of the nodule may be indicated, especially if there are other underlying features of malignancy.

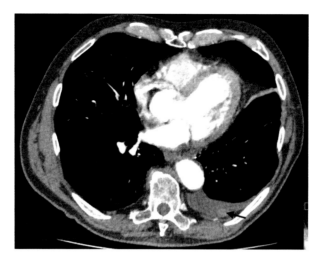

Figure 18.3 CT scan image of the pleural-based abnormality (arrow).

If SFTP is suspected, it is usually not PET avid. A preoperative biopsy is not indicated to determine the malignant potential, as biopsy has been shown to have low sensitivity, and the result may not correlate with the histology of the entire resected nodule. Tumour seeding into the pleural space or tract has been reported after biopsy, but the risk is thought to be low (4). If SFTP is suspected, surgical resection provides a diagnostic and potentially curative procedure.

The chest pain, pleural plaques, history of asbestos exposure and the pleural effusion, albeit low volume, raised the suspicion of possible underlying malignant mesothelioma. An ultrasound-guided pleural biopsy was therefore performed. The histology showed atypical mesothelial proliferation, and although there was minimal invasion noted on the sample, the findings were suspicious for epithelioid or biphasic mesothelioma. The diagnosis of mesothelioma was ratified during discussion with the multidisciplinary team.

c) What is the best way of managing a solitary fibrous tumour of the pleura?

Management of SFTP can include resection, chemotherapy and radiotherapy. However, the evidence base for SFTP management is limited and there is therefore no consensus guideline on management. If the patient is a surgical candidate, then surgical resection is usually offered as a diagnostic and potentially curative procedure. However, smaller lesions (<4 cm) can be monitored radiologically only as the chances of malignant involvement tends to be lower. Given that SFTP may recur after resection, and that 23% of first recurrences occur after 5 years, follow-up is recommended radiologically at 3, 6 and 12 months after diagnosis or resection, and yearly thereafter for 10 years (2). Where possible, MRI is useful for imaging surveillance due to the decreased radiation exposure associated with MRI when compared to CT scan (2).

d) What is the best way of managing localised mesothelioma?

Guidelines on optimal management in this scenario vary. The American Society of Clinical Oncology guidelines published in 2018 recommends maximal surgical cytoreduction in selected patients with early-stage non-sarcomatoid mesothelioma, as part of multimodality treatment, while the British Thoracic Society guidelines published in the same year recommend surgery only as part of research trials (5, 6).

In this case, this patient was referred for systemic therapy for his malignant pleural mesothelioma and started on palliative chemotherapy.

## KEY POINTS

- A biopsy is not recommended in suspected SFTP because of the low sensitivity and potential different histology from that of the resected nodule.
- SFTP are usually benign and surgery is potentially curative, however, radiological surveillance is recommended for up to 10 years after diagnosis/resection because of the risk of malignancy/recurrence.
- There is controversy on the best way to manage localised malignant pleural mesothelioma, with American guidelines recommending multimodality treatment including surgery, and British guidelines recommending surgery only as part of research trials.

## REFERENCES

1. Sureka B, Thukral BB, Mittal MK, Mittal A, Sinha M. Radiological review of pleural tumors. *Indian J Radiol Imaging*. 2013;23(4):313–20.
2. Mercer RM, Wigston C, Banka R, Cardillo G, Benamore R, Nicholson AG, et al. Management of solitary fibrous tumours of the pleura: A systematic review and meta-analysis. *ERJ Open Research*. 2020 July;6(3):00055-2020.
3. Luciano C, Francesco A, Giovanni V, Federica S. Cesare F. CT signs, patterns and differential diagnosis of solitary fibrous tumors of the pleura. *J Thorac Dis*. 2010 March;2(1):21–5.
4. Scarsbrook AF, Evans AL, Slade M, Gleeson FV. Recurrent solitary fibrous tumour of the pleura due to tumour seeding following ultrasound-guided transthoracic biopsy. *Clin Radiol*. 2005 January;60(1):130–2.
5. Kindler HL, Ismaila N, Armato SG, Bueno R, Hesdorffer M, Jahan T, et al. Treatment of malignant pleural mesothelioma: American Society of Clinical Oncology clinical practice guideline. *Journal of Clinical Oncology*. 2018 May;36(13):1343–73.
6. Woolhouse I, Bishop L, Darlison L, De Fonseka D, Edey A, Edwards J, et al. British thoracic society guideline for the investigation and management of malignant pleural mesothelioma. *Thorax*. 2018 March;73(Suppl 1):i1–30.

# 19

# Pneumothorax in chronic lung disease

BEENISH IQBAL

A 78-year-old lady with end-stage idiopathic pulmonary fibrosis (IPF) and COPD on long-term oxygen therapy at 2 L/min presented to the emergency department with sudden onset right-sided chest pain and worsening breathlessness. Before admission, she had a poor exercise tolerance that was limited to a few yards only on the flat.

On presentation, she was in severe respiratory distress with the following observations: pulse rate 105/min, BP 210/120 mmHg, RR 30/min, saturation 87% on 15 L/min $O_2$ via non-rebreather oxygen reservoir mask. On examination, there were absent breath sounds on the right side and hyper-resonant percussion notes. An urgent chest X-ray (CXR) was conducted (Figure 19.1).

a) What is the diagnosis based on the clinical presentation and the CXR?

The patient has acute right-sided secondary spontaneous pneumothorax (SSP) due to underlying COPD and IPF.

SSP is defined as a collection of air between parietal and visceral pleura in patients with underlying lung disease or >50 years of age with significant smoking history (1). Consequently, these patients have a high symptom burden, sometimes out of proportion to the size of the pneumothorax. It is estimated that about 60% of pneumothorax admissions are due to SSP (2). These patients are usually sicker than patients with primary spontaneous pneumothorax (PSP), which occurs in a younger population with no under-lying lung disease. Hence, there is a lower threshold for intervention in SSP if symptomatic, irrespective of the size of the pneumothorax.

A subsequent CT chest confirmed the findings (Figure 19.2). She underwent an emergency 12Fr intercostal chest drain insertion connected to an underwater

DOI: 10.1201/9781003081630-19

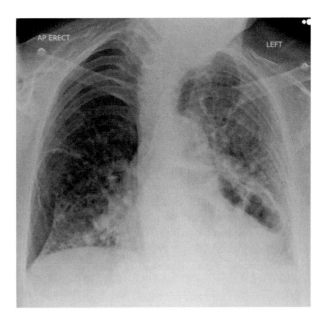

Figure 19.1 Chest X-ray showing a moderate to large, right-sided basal pneumothorax. There is visible underlying reticular shadowing with rib crowding showing fibrosis.

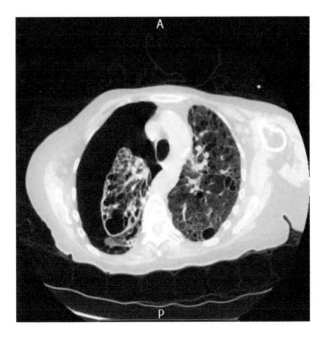

Figure 19.2 Large right-sided pneumothorax with underlying emphysema and fibrosis.

seal that resulted in immediate symptomatic improvement and reduction in oxygen requirement. A digital suction device was used for accurate air leak measurement, demonstrating an air leak of 1 L/min.

Despite showing initial improvement, the pneumothorax persisted after 4–5 days of chest drainage, with a large air leak, and a repeat CXR was conducted (Figure 19.3).

b) What is the likely explanation for her current clinical condition and how it should be managed?

This is a case of non-resolving pneumothorax with persistent air leak (PAL), which is defined as an ongoing air leak after 5–7 days of chest drain insertion to treat pneumothorax. This is usually due to an alveolar/bronchopleural fistulous connection that causes air to flow from the lung to the pleural space. These can be divided into those where an air leak occurs on forced expiration, simple expiration, inspiration or occur continuously, the latter being predictive of larger air leaks (3).

Patients with PAL who are deemed fit for invasive treatment options should be discussed with thoracic surgeons for consideration of surgical treatment with either open thoracotomy or video-assisted thoracoscopic surgery (VATS) involving resection of the diseased lung/pleura with or without pleurodesis (4). There is limited evidence on surgical outcomes of these patients and an overall mortality up to 5% has been noted in retrospective case series (5), with some smaller studies suggesting worse outcomes in interstitial lung disease (ILD) patients than COPD (6). As most such patients are considered high-risk for invasive treatment, a more pragmatic approach with conservative and non-invasive options is often adopted.

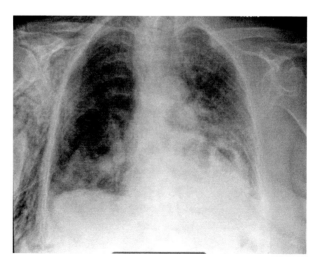

Figure 19.3 Repeat CXR showing chest drain in situ with significant subcutaneous emphysema.

Due to a poor functional baseline and severe underlying lung disease, she was not deemed suitable for surgical treatment. A decision was made to treat her non-surgically.

c) What are the treatment options for conservative (non-surgical) management of PAL?

Observational data suggests that PAL resolves in 14 days in 79% of patients of SSP without further intervention (7) (beyond the initial chest drainage). However, for those who continue to have ongoing air leaks, other management options are as follows (2,8):

- *Large bore chest drain with/without ambulatory Heimlich valve device*: A chest drain with a larger diameter allows a larger volume of airflow. This is not only better in managing the air leaking through the pleural space but also in improving/avoiding extra air escaping into the subcutaneous tissue causing subcutaneous emphysema. In some cases, the large bore tube alone is sufficient to provide drainage while the pleural breach undergoes healing. However, this can be associated with prolonged hospital stay (8)

  This problem can be addressed by attaching the drain to an ambulatory one-way Heimlich valve, allowing mobilisation and potential discharge of the patient (2). This is more safely delivered using larger bore drains (18F and above), as they are less likely to block compared to smaller bore drains. Case series suggest that this treatment can shorten hospital stay with PAL by 46% (9). However, this treatment approach requires close follow-up and easy access to hospital services if complications (blockage, valve failure, displacement, infection) arise.

- *Thoracic suction via the chest drain*: Application of negative suction to the chest drainage system to allow 'quicker' resolution of pneumothorax has been in use for a long time. However, it has very little evidence base and multiple studies have failed to prove its superiority over passive drainage using an underwater seal (10,11) Some studies show harm in post-operative patients with severe emphysema (7). The British Thoracic Society (BTS) guidelines do not advocate the routine use of thoracic suction for pneumothorax (1).

  Thoracic suction used for this purpose is high volume and low pressure and delivered either by traditional wall suction or newer digital suction devices. The range of suction pressure is also debatable, ranging from −0.5 kPa to −2.0 kPa (or equivalent in mmHg or cmH$_2$O), mainly based on post-surgical patient data (10).

- *Chemical pleurodesis*: Chemical pleurodesis involves the use of sclerosants such as sterile-graded talc and doxycycline to induce inflammation between the parietal and visceral pleura to promote obliteration of the pleural space. However, this treatment requires apposition between the parietal and visceral pleural surfaces, which may not be present in pneumothorax with PAL. A small study has shown promising results with a 94% success rate in such patients using talc via thoracoscopy or chest drain; however, there was no control group and resolution of PAL took up to 12 days (12). Nevertheless, the use of chemical pleurodesis has been acknowledged by current guidelines for recurrence prevention in patients with SSP who are not fit for surgical intervention (1).

- *Autologous blood patch pleurodesis (ABP)*: Blood patch pleurodesis has been postulated to help with the healing of bronchopleural fistula leading to PAL by both forming a clot over the fistula and inducing a pleurodesis. A variable dose of blood ranging between 50 and 120 ml has been used in small studies (8). There are concerns about the potential complication of pleural infection with the use of ABP. A recent systematic review has shown that although ABP is safe in PAL with SSP, the overall success is <50% if PAL is >5 days. The risk of infection was about 9% in two studies (13). ABP should therefore be considered after weighing the risks versus benefits for each patient.
- *Endobronchial valves (EBVs)*: Endobronchial valves are one-way valves that are used to achieve bronchoscopic lung volume reduction in emphysema with profound gas trapping. They are inserted through the bronchoscope into lobar, segmental or subsegmental bronchi to occlude the airway-supplying emphysematous lung. They have been used in PAL to occlude the airway feeding the bronchopleural fistula and to allow pneumothorax resolution. However, the procedure involves multiple sessions to identify sites of leakage (which is not always possible) and for successful deployment of the EBV, and usually involves sedation and sometimes general anaesthetic. The success rate reported has been variable in small studies of highly selected patients (8).

The patient underwent a further large bore 26Fr chest drain insertion, and digital suction was used up to –1.5 kPa. There was slow improvement in the pneumothorax and air leak with radiological resolution of pneumothorax on subsequent imaging. However, clamping trials under controlled conditions demonstrated a recurrence of pneumothorax.

A blood patch pleurodesis was therefore conducted (2 ml/kg of autologous blood), but it was unsuccessful. Over a period of days, the air leak started slowly improving, followed by slowly reducing thoracic suction and careful monitoring. Once the thoracic suction was stopped and the air leak was small, i.e. 100–200 ml/min, the chest drain was connected to an ambulatory Heimlich valve and the patient was monitored for 48 h in hospital while mobilising. She remained stable and was discharged home with the chest drain and Heimlich valve in situ, with once-weekly pleural follow-up. Four weeks after discharge, the pneumothorax had completely resolved with no ongoing air leak. A clamping trial was conducted and demonstrated no evidence of recurrence on the thoracic CT scan (Figures 19.4 and 19.5). The chest drain was safely removed and the patient remained well with no further recurrence.

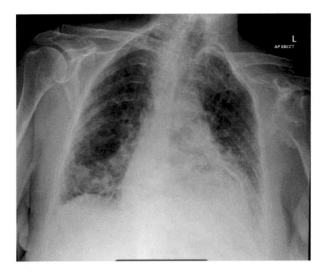

Figure 19.4 Resolution of right-sided pneumothorax on CXR.

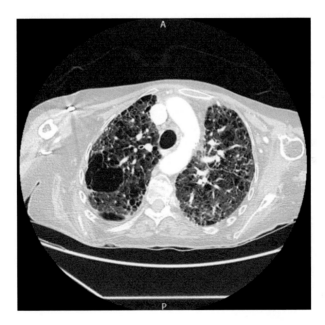

Figure 19.5 Resolution of right-sided pneumothorax on CT scan.

## KEY POINTS

- Secondary pneumothorax is often associated with significant symptoms and physiological compromise, and the intervention threshold should be lower, even in those with small pneumothoraces.
- Prolonged air leak is more common in secondary pneumothorax than with primary disease.
- Treatment options should always include a discussion to assess surgical suitability, with thoracic surgical intervention the best treatment option for patients who are fit enough.
- In those unable to undergo surgery, ambulatory treatment and allowing healing over time, blood patch pleurodesis, talc pleurodesis, and endobronchial valves can be considered.

## REFERENCES

1. MacDuff A, Arnold A, Harvey J; BTS Pleural Disease Guideline Group. Management of spontaneous pneumothorax: British Thoracic Society pleural disease guideline 2010. *Thorax* 2010; 65 (Supplement 2): i18–i31.
2. Walker SP, Keenan E, Bintcliffe O, et al. Ambulatory management of secondary spontaneous pneumothorax: A randomised controlled trial. *Eur Respir J* 2021; 57(6): 2003375.
3. Dugan KC, Laxmanan B, Murgu S, Hogarth DK. Management of persistent air leaks. *Chest* 2017; 152(2): 417–423.
4. Porcel JM, Lee P. Thoracoscopy for spontaneous pneumothorax. *J Clin Med* 2021; 10(17): 3835.
5. Zhang Y, Jiang G, Chen C, Ding J, Zhu Y, Xu Z. Surgical management of secondary spontaneous pneumothorax in elderly patients with chronic obstructive pulmonary disease: Retrospective series of 107 patients. *Thorac Cardiovasc Surg* 2009; 57(6): 347–352.
6. Nakajima J, Takamoto S, Murakawa T, Fukami T, Yoshida Y, Kusakabe M. Outcome of thoracoscopic management of secondary pneumothorax in patients with COPD and interstitial pulmonary fibrosis. *Surg Endosc* 2009; 23(7): 1536–1540.
7. Chee CBE, Abisheganaden J, Yeo JK, et al. Persistent air-leak in spontaneous pneumothorax-clinical course and outcome. *Respir Med* 1998; 92(5): 757–761.
8. Nava GW, Walker SP. Management of the secondary spontaneous pneumothorax. Current guidance, controversies and recent advances. *J Clin Med* 2022; 11(5): 1173.
9. McKenna RJ Jr, Fischel RJ, Brenner M, Gelb AF. Use of Heimlich valve to shorten hospital stay after lung reduction surgery for emphysema. *Ann Thorac Surg* 1996; 61(4): 1115–1117.

10. Brunelli A, Salati M, Pompili C, Refai M, Sabbatini A. Regulated tailored suction vs. regulated seal: A prospective randomised trial on air leak duration. *Eur J Cardio Thorac Surg* 2013; 43(5): 899–904.
11. So SY, Yu DY. Catheter drainage of spontaneous pneumothorax: Suction or no suction, early or late removal? *Thorax* 1982; 37(1): 46–48.
12. Watanabe T, Fukai I, Okuda K, et al. Talc pleurodesis for secondary pneumothorax in elderly patients with persistent air leak. *J Thorac Dis* 2019; 11(1): 171–176.
13. Shafiq M, Banka R, Bain PA, Mahmood K, Rahman NM, Cheng G. Autologous blood patch for persistent air leak following secondary spontaneous pneumothorax: A systematic review. *J Bronchol Interv Pulmonol* 2023;30(1):70–75.

# 20

# Air in the wrong place

ROB HALLIFAX

A 54-year-old man of British Asian origin presented to hospital with a 4-day history of cough, change in taste and breathlessness in January 2021. He was confirmed COVID-19 positive on PCR testing. Usually fit and well, his past medical history included hypertension and obesity.

On admission to hospital, his oxygen saturations were 80% on air and he was tachypnoeic with a respiratory rate of 30 breaths per minute. The patient was admitted to the respiratory ward. Oxygen therapy, dexamethasone and remdesivir were administered (as constituted standard care at the time). He became increasingly symptomatic with hypoxaemic respiratory failure (type 1). Continuous positive airway pressure (CPAP) therapy was initiated with awake proning.

Unfortunately, after 2 days the oxygen requirement increased further and he had increasingly laboured breathing. Clinically, on examination, there was now significant subcutaneous emphysema. Chest computed tomography (CT) scanning revealed worsening COVID-19 pneumonitis and extensive pneumomediastinum (Figure 20.1).

a) What is the incidence of pneumomediastinum and pneumothorax associated with COVID-19 pneumonitis?

There are multiple small case reports of pneumothorax in patients with COVID-19 pneumonitis. The best data comes from two large collaborative multi-centre retrospective series in the UK.

Martinelli et al. reported on 71 patients from 16 UK hospitals between March and June 2020 (1). Sixty had pneumothoraces (six with concurrent pneumomediastinum) and 11 had pneumomediastinum alone. Although COVID-19 patient data were not available for all hospitals, 60 cases were identified in centres with an estimated 6,574 COVID-19 admissions, giving an estimated incidence of 0.91%.

DOI: 10.1201/9781003081630-20

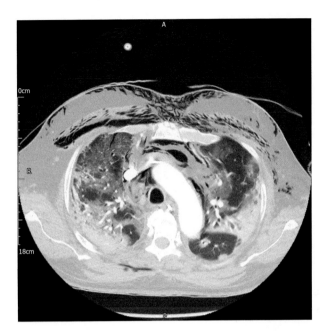

Figure 20.1 Computed tomography (CT) scan for the chest showing extensive anterior subcutaneous emphysema and pneumomediastinum.

Melhorn et al. compiled data from 53 UK hospitals including 377 cases of pneumomediastinum from 58,484 COVID-19–positive inpatients between September 2020 and February 2021, giving an incidence of 0.64% (2). Pneumothorax was seen concurrently in 154/377 patients (40.8%) and subcutaneous emphysema was seen in 280/377 patients (74.3%).

Unfortunately, the patient continued to deteriorate despite CPAP, with increased $O_2$ requirement, and was tiring. The left-sided pneumothorax enlarged on subsequent chest radiology. He was intubated and admitted to the intensive care unit (ICU). No intercostal drain insertion was required and the pneumothorax did not expand in size despite ventilation. Four weeks later, whilst still ventilated, oxygen requirements began to increase. Chest radiography showed a significant left-sided pneumothorax (Figure 20.2), and a left-sided chest tube was inserted.

b) What is the mechanism of pneumomediastinum (and/or pneumothorax) and its association with high inspiratory pressures (e.g. CPAP or invasive ventilation)?

The mechanism of formation of pneumomediastinum is thought to be the 'Macklin effect' (3). Macklin describes pneumomediastinum as secondary to the rupture of marginal alveoli due to a markedly increased pressure gradient between the alveolus and the interstitial space. After rupture of the alveolus, air dissects along the sheaths of the bronchovascular bundles

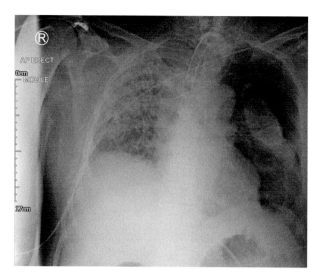

Figure 20.2 Chest radiography showing left-sided pneumothorax.

medially towards the mediastinum. In severe cases, the air can decompress from the mediastinum along cervical fascial planes into the subcutaneous tissues of the chest wall, neck or face. In addition, air may rupture through the thin mediastinal pleural surface into the pleural space causing unilateral or bilateral pneumothoraces.

The increased pressure provided by CPAP or invasive ventilation could potentially drive the increased pressure gradient between the alveolar and interstitial spaces leading to pneumomediastinum. However, pneumomediastinum appears to occur in the context of severe COVID-19 infection, which then requires a high degree of respiratory support, i.e. the positive pressures used are not in themselves causative. It is possible that the severity of the underlying parenchymal disease itself seen in COVID-19, with the associated inflammation of the alveolar-interstitial membrane, is the risk factor for the formation of the pneumomediastinum (2).

In the multi-centre series of 377 pneumomediastinum cases, 205 patients (54.4%) were not invasively ventilated at the point the diagnosis of pneumomediastinum was made (2). Therefore, invasive ventilation was not a likely precursor of pneumomediastinum for the majority of patients. The severity of the disease was demonstrated with a mortality rate of 51.7% (195/377) in these patients (2).

Once the left-sided pneumothorax had resolved, the chest drain was removed. He had a long ICU stay and was ventilated for a further 2 months, with multiple further complications including acute renal failure (requiring haemofiltration) and multiple ventilator-associated pneumonias.

c) Should the management of COVID-19 be altered once pneumomediastinum has been identified?

Theoretically, ongoing positive pressure could exacerbate pneumomediastinum. However, in this patient population with severe COVID-19 pneumonitis, weaning to lower pressures may not be feasible. In the absence of randomised controlled trial data, the multi-centre series of 377 pneumomediastinum cases reported 93 patients eligible for invasive ventilation at the time of diagnosis of pneumomediastinum were on CPAP. Fifty (53.8%) of these patients were switched immediately on diagnosis to oxygen or high-flow oxygen therapy and 43 continued CPAP. These two groups were similarly matched by demographics and fractional inspired oxygen and there was no difference in survival according to whether the patient was switched to high-flow oxygen or not (2).

Once weaned off invasive ventilation, the patient was stepped down to the respiratory ward for further care and rehabilitation. He was initially discharged with home oxygen. He has since been reviewed in the pneumothorax and post-COVID clinics and has made a good recovery. Home oxygen is no longer required, and he continues to improve his mobility and exercise capacity. Follow-up CT scanning showed persistent bilateral subpleural reticulation and septal thickening, with an upper zone predominance, associated architectural distortion and traction bronchiectasis, in keeping with post–COVID-19 pulmonary fibrosis.

d) What are the long-term implications of pneumothorax or pneumomediastinum with COVID-19?

There are no long-term data on the risk of recurrent spontaneous pneumothorax or pneumomediastinum in patients who experienced them in the context of COVID-19 pneumonitis. Large-scale national dataset studies are required to determine the ongoing risk of future episodes and complications.

The patient has not suffered from any further pneumothoraces or pneumomediastinum episodes but does have ongoing breathlessness. His lung function tests show a forced expiratory volume in 1 second (FEV1) 1.9 L (60%), forced vital capacity (FVC) 2.3 L (58%), giving a ratio of 81%. His TLCO was 41% but corrected for KCO at 100% likely due to his underlying pulmonary fibrosis.

## KEY POINTS

- Pneumothorax and pneumomediastinum are uncommon but significant complications of COVID-19 pneumothorax, with incidences of 0.91% and 0.64% of hospitalised patients, respectively.
- Pneumothorax and pneumomediastinum are associated with severe COVID-19 disease. Iatrogenic high inspiratory pressures do not seem to be a prerequisite for their formation.

- Practically, positive pressure should be weaned, if possible, but continued positive pressure ventilation if required for disease severity does not appear to be detrimental.
- The long-term risk of further spontaneous pneumothorax or pneumomediastinum is not known.

## REFERENCES

1. Martinelli AW, Ingle T, Newman J, Nadeem I, Jackson K, Lane ND, et al. COVID-19 and pneumothorax: A multicentre retrospective case series. *Eur Respir J* 2020;56(5):2002697.
2. Melhorn J, Achaiah A, Conway FM, Thompson EMF, Skyllberg EW, Durrant J, et al. Pneumomediastinum in COVID-19: A phenotype of severe COVID-19 pneumonitis? The results of the United Kingdom (POETIC) survey. *Eur Respir J* 2022;60(3):2102522.
3. Macklin MT, Macklin CC. Malignant interstitial emphysema of the lungs and mediastinum as an important occult complication in many respiratory diseases and other conditions: An interpretation of the clinical literature in the light of laboratory experiment. *Medicine* 1944;23(4):281–358.

# 21

# Recurrent chest pain in a young woman

BEENISH IQBAL

A 34-year-old lady presented to the pleural outpatient clinic with 2–3 weeks of right-sided chest pain, breathlessness and a new moderate right pleural effusion on chest X-ray (Figure 21.1). She was otherwise fit and well, and a never smoker. Her only past medical history was primary infertility for which she was undergoing investigations. Her observations were within normal range and her blood tests were unremarkable.

A thoracic ultrasound was conducted in the clinic that confirmed the presence of a large, right-sided pleural effusion (Figure 21.2).

A diagnostic and therapeutic pleural aspiration was conducted under ultrasound guidance. Fluid was blood-stained, exudative with protein 37 g/dl, LDH 250 IU/L and glucose 4.8 mmol/L. Pleural fluid cytology showed mixed inflammatory cells with eosinophilic predominance. Pleural fluid microscopy, culture and sensitivity (MC&S) were negative for bacteria including acid-fast bacillus (AFB).

a) What is the differential diagnosis?

The differential diagnosis of an eosinophilic effusion is broad and the commonest causes include malignancy (26%), idiopathic (25%), parapneumonic (13%), air or blood in pleural space (13%), tuberculosis (7%), and other (6%) including drug-induced and autoimmune causes (1). A systematic approach is needed to narrow the differentials and reach the correct diagnosis.

She had no red-flag features of malignancy and a CT of the chest, abdomen, and pelvis showed right-sided pleural effusion with normal underlying pleura, and small volume ascites but no overt malignancy. There were no preceding infective symptoms before this presentation and no lung parenchymal

DOI: 10.1201/9781003081630-21

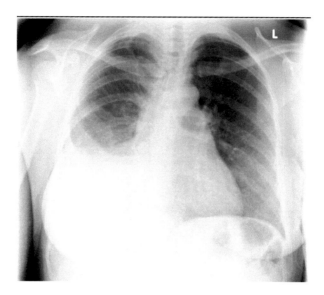

Figure 21.1 Chest radiograph showing the presence of right-sided moderate pleural effusion.

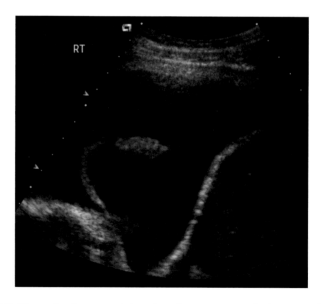

Figure 21.2 Thoracic ultrasound showing the presence of a large, right-sided, non-septated, non-echogenic pleural effusion.

infiltrates on CT chest so a parapneumonic effusion was unlikely. Although the effusion was blood-stained, she had no trauma before this and there was no evidence of pneumothorax on imaging. She was not started on any medications including antibiotics prior to this illness so drug-induced cause was unlikely. Her autoimmune profile and parasitic screening were normal.

A local anaesthetic thoracoscopy was performed to obtain pleural biopsies. At this examination, the parietal and visceral pleura were macroscopically normal with small pleural effusion. A few cystic lesions were found on the diaphragmatic pleural surface that were biopsied (Figures 21.3 and 21.4).

An MRI thorax also showed cystic lesions in the costophrenic angle near the diaphragm (Figure 21.5).

The histopathology of the lesions and the MRI thorax were in keeping with thoracic endometriosis. An MRI pelvis showed concurrent pelvic endometriosis that was considered the likely cause of her primary infertility.

b) What is thoracic endometriosis?

Endometriosis is a chronic condition that is characterised by the growth of endometrial (uterine) tissue outside the uterine cavity and affects 10% of women in their reproductive age. Thoracic endometriosis occurs due to the deposition of endometrial tissue in the thoracic cavity, particularly the lung, pleura and diaphragm, and it is the most common extra-abdominopelvic site for endometriosis (2).

Thoracic endometriosis is considered a syndrome with multiple presentations ranging from catamenial pneumothorax (80%), catamenial haemothorax (14%), catamenial haemoptysis (5%), rarely diaphragmatic

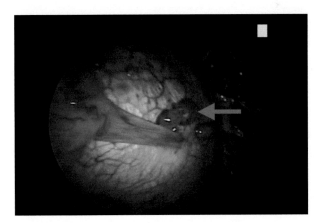

Figure 21.3 Thoracoscopic image showing the presence of cystic lesions on the diaphragmatic pleural surface (blue arrow).

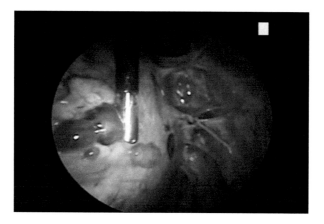

Figure 21.4 Thoracoscopic image demonstrating biopsy of cystic lesion on diaphragmatic pleural surface.

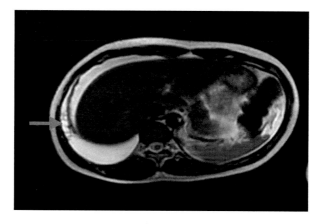

Figure 21.5 An axial image of MRI thorax showing cystic lesions near the costophrenic surface of the diaphragm (blue arrow).

rupture and lung nodules (2, 3). The pathophysiology of thoracic endometriosis is not fully understood but retrograde menstruation theory (with endometrial tissue escaping into the peritoneum via the fallopian tube during menstruation), lymphatic and haematogenous spread are considered the most likely mechanisms. The disease is right-sided in 92% of cases (2).

Many patients with thoracic endometriosis are asymptomatic. If symptomatic, the severity and nature of symptoms depend on the location of endometrial tissue within the thoracic cavity. Cyclical catamenial symptoms

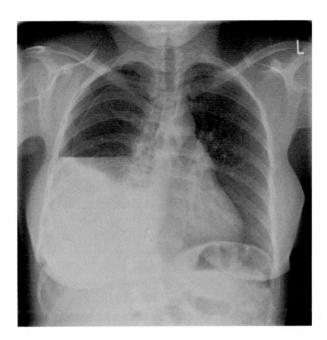

Figure 21.6 Chest X-ray showing the presence of a large, right-sided hydropneumothorax.

like chest pain, cough, breathlessness and shoulder tip pain due to diaphragmatic lesions can occur 24 h before and up to 72 h after the onset of menstruation (3).

One month later, she presented to the emergency department with sudden worsening of right-sided chest pain. A chest X-ray was conducted (Figure 21.6).

She started her menstruation 2 days before this presentation and a diagnosis of catamenial haemopneumothorax was made. She was treated with chest drain insertion for the haemopneumothorax and adequate analgesia was administered to manage the chest pain. She continued to have recurrent right-sided pleural effusion with increasing chest pain during menstruation.

c) How do you diagnose and manage thoracic endometriosis?

There is no single test to diagnose thoracic endometriosis (TE) and a strong clinical suspicion remains the key to diagnosis. A chest X-ray can detect pneumothorax and pleural effusion but a suggestive history of TE with clinical symptoms should prompt further chest imaging with CT or MRI. An MRI thorax during menstruation is helpful to delineate endometrial deposits, especially diaphragmatic, with a sensitivity of 78%–83% for the latter but poor specificity (4). The aim should be to obtain tissue diagnosis for confirmation.

The management of TE is based on the severity of symptoms and a multidisciplinary team approach is required, including a gynaecologist, chest physician, radiologist and surgeon. The first-line treatment is with medical therapy to block the hypothalamic–pituitary–ovarian axis and to stop the proliferation of endometrial tissue by suppressing ovarian hormone production. If medical management is not effective, surgical treatment is considered (3).

For medical treatment, the commonly used hormonal therapy is gonadotropin-releasing hormone (GnRH) agonists. This treatment effectively causes hypogonadotropic hypogonadism and amenorrhoea, thus controlling the symptoms. However, the discontinuation of GnRH agonists can lead to higher recurrence rates, and long-term treatment can cause menopause-like symptoms and osteoporosis (5). Other medications include oral contraceptives, progestins, danazol and aromatase inhibitors. Treatment is usually given for 6–12 months with regular assessments.

For refractory and recurrent severe cases, surgical treatment is indicated, which requires careful case-by-case discussion, as most patients have both thoracic and pelvic endometriosis and a concomitant treatment is needed in about 44% of cases (3, 6). Video-assisted thoracoscopic surgery (VATS) is considered a gold-standard technique for pleural and diaphragmatic lesions. The surgery includes pleurectomy with or without chemical pleurodesis for the pleural lesions. Diaphragmatic deposits are noted in 84% of patients during surgery (6) and are treated with excision followed by coagulation with a $CO_2$ laser or electrocautery. Adjuvant hormonal therapy is given in almost all cases after surgery to reduce the chances of recurrence, which occurs in about 27% of cases (6).

The patient was treated with GnRH analogues for more than 6 months, but her symptoms continued. She underwent VATS pleurectomy and pleurodesis for pleural disease, and the pelvic endometriosis was treated laparoscopically. She was given adjuvant GnRH analogues for a few months and gradually withdrawn with careful monitoring for recurrence. She was followed up for 5 years with no recurrence of her pleural disease.

## KEY POINTS

- Symptoms of thoracic endometriosis are non-specific, hence a detailed clinical history and a high degree of clinical suspicion are required.
- Medical management forms the first line of treatment.
- Definitive treatment involves combined video laparoscopy and video-assisted thoracoscopic surgery.
- Post-operative hormonal therapy may occasionally be needed to prevent further recurrence.

# REFERENCES

1. Oba Y, Abu-Salah T. The prevalence and diagnostic significance of eosinophilic pleural effusions: A meta-analysis and systematic review. *Respiration*. 2012;83(3):198–208.
2. Velagapudi RK, Egan JP. Thoracic endometriosis: A clinical review and update of current and evolving diagnostic and therapeutic techniques. *Curr Pulmonol Rep*. 2021;10(1):22–9.
3. Nezhat C, Lindheim SR, Backhus L, Vu M, Vang N, Nezhat A, et al. Thoracic endometriosis syndrome: A review of diagnosis and management. *JSLS*. 2019;23(3): e2019.00029.
4. Rousset P, Gregory J, Rousset-Jablonski C, Hugon-Rodin J, Regnard JF, Chapron C, et al. MR diagnosis of diaphragmatic endometriosis. *Eur Radiol*. 2016;26(11):3968–77.
5. McKee DC, Mansour T, Wasson MN. Thoracic and diaphragmatic endometriosis: An overview of diagnosis and surgical treatment. *Curr Opin Obstet Gynecol*. 2022;34(4):204–9.
6. Ciriaco P, Muriana P, Lembo R, Carretta A, Negri G. Treatment of thoracic endometriosis syndrome: A meta-analysis and review. *Ann Thorac Surg*. 2022;113(1):324–36.

# An interesting case of recurrent pneumothoraces

ROB HALLIFAX

A 24-year-old British woman was seen in the Oxford pneumothorax clinic having 3 weeks previously her second right-sided primary spontaneous pneumothorax (PSP). Her first episode, 2 years ago, was managed conservatively, but on this occasion, she was managed with a chest tube as an inpatient after a failed needle aspiration. She was a never smoker and did not have any other past medical history. There was no temporal association between her menstrual cycle and pneumothorax episodes.

She attends clinic for follow-up. On further questioning, her mother had also suffered from recurrent pneumothoraces in her early 30s and eventually had thoracic surgery for recurrence prevention.

a. How common is familial pneumothorax?

A significant proportion of patients with PSP will report a family history. This is often quoted as ~10% based on two small retrospective studies. The first (from 1991) was a study of males who served in the Israel Defense Forces, in which 33 of 286 patients surveyed reported a family history of PSP (1). Of these 33, family pedigrees for 15 families were examined (along with constructed pedigrees from an available literature search). The pattern of inheritance was complex, but the authors concluded that it was most likely that PSP predisposition is due to more than one gene (1). The second was an analysis of 102 Chinese patients with sporadic and familial isolated PSP (2) in which 10 patients reported a strong family history. More recently, however, a large randomised controlled trial of ambulatory management of PSP has replicated this figure of 10% of patients having a first-degree relative with pneumothorax (3).

b. What types of familial conditions are associated with spontaneous pneumothorax?

Conditions associated with pneumothorax can be categorised into those resulting from tumour suppressor genes and those with defects in the

DOI: 10.1201/9781003081630-22

extracellular matrix (4). The two classic conditions related to tumour suppressor genes are Birt–Hogg–Dubé (BHD) syndrome and tuberous sclerosis complex (TSC)/lymphangioleiomyomatosis (LAM). BHD is an autosomal dominant condition caused by heterozygous mutations in FLCN, which encode folliculin (5). LAM is a progressive lung disease which occurs (almost entirely) in young females (6) and involves infiltration of the alveolar septa with smooth muscle-like 'LAM cells' and the development of cysts (7). LAM can occur sporadically but also in association with TSC. TSC is an autosomal dominant (AD) condition caused by germline loss-of-function mutations in TSC1 (encoding hamartin) or TSC2 (encoding tuberin) (8, 9).

Conditions with defects in the extracellular matrix include Marfan syndrome, Loeys–Dietz and vascular Ehlers–Danlos syndrome. Marfan syndrome is an AD condition caused by mutations in FBN1 which encodes fibrillin 1. Loeys–Dietz syndrome is an AD genetic disorder caused by mutations in genes which encode parts of the TGF-β signalling pathway. Ehlers–Danlos syndrome (EDS) is a family of connective disorders mostly resulting from mutations in collagen pathways. Only the vascular subtype (type IV), vEDS, is associated with pneumothorax. vEDS is an AD genetic disorder of the COL3A1 gene coding for type III collagen (10).

On examination, the patient was tall and thin but did not have translucent skin, pectus excavatum or a longer arm span than height. She did not have excessively flexible joints. However, she did have small, firm, white papules on her nose, cheeks and upper chest, consistent with fibrofolliculomas.

c. What features on examination could suggest a familial condition?

Patients with BHD may have fibrofolliculomas, characteristic findings on their skin (hamartomas of hair follicles) which are small, dome-shaped papules typically on the face, neck, chest, back and arms. Skin tags are also occasionally seen.

If the patient has LAM that is associated with TSC, skin findings may include hypopigmented macules (ash leaf spots), facial angiofibromas and Shagreen patches. LAM patients can also present with breathlessness and wheezing due to obstructive lung disease from pulmonary interstitial disease. Non-pulmonary findings (of TSC) include renal cysts or carcinoma, cardiac arrhythmias, retinal hamartomas and cortical dysplasia (tubers).

The classic Marfan syndrome phenotype is tall, thin body habitus, with long limbs resulting in decreased upper segment to lower segment ratio (and wider arm span than height), long thin fingers (arachnodactyly), chest wall deformity, scoliosis, lens dislocation (ectopia lentis), and aortic dilation (11). The current diagnostic criteria have aortic root aneurysm and ectopia lentis as cardinal features. In the absence of any family history, the presence of these two features is sufficient for the unequivocal diagnosis of Marfan syndrome. In the absence of one of these two cardinal features, the presence of an FBN1 mutation or positive systemic score is required. Systemic features do include pneumothorax

(2 points), but ≥7 points are required, so pneumothorax alone without other features is not sufficient (12). Pneumothorax does appear to be more common in patients with Marfan syndrome than in the general population.

Pneumothorax does occasionally occur in patients with Loeys–Dietz syndrome (11). Patients classically have bifid uvula or cleft palate, retrognathia, joint laxity or contractures, scoliosis, arachnodactyly, and pectus excavatum on examination. The skin may be translucent in appearance with easy bruising. Other common features are vascular abnormalities (arterial aneurysms or dissections) and uterine rupture (during pregnancy) (13).

In vEDS, patients may have micrognathia with thin lips and nose, and prominent eyes. Skin is often translucent with visible veins. Orthopaedic complications include clubfoot, congenital hip dislocation and tendon rupture (14). Serious (and potentially fatal) complications include aneurysms, dissection and rupture of arteries, uterus and intestines. (14).

After elucidating a strong family history and finding features on examination in keeping with BHD, a chest computed tomography (CT) scan is performed to look for pulmonary abnormalities.

d. Can imaging be useful in screening for familial conditions?

Pulmonary cysts are very common in BHD. The cysts are irregular in shape and tend to have a basal predominance and tend to be subpleural including paramediastinal (15, 16) (Figure 22.1). Renal cysts are common in BHD and there is an increased risk of renal cancers. Therefore, all patients should have renal MRI or ultrasound at diagnosis of BHD and then be scheduled for regular (annual) screening.

In LAM, the cysts tend to be smaller, round in shape and fewer in number than BHD (16). The dominant finding in LAM is interstitial changes which can progress and cause obstructive lung disease. Treatments are available to slow the rate of decline of lung function (e.g. mTORC1 inhibitor, sirolimus) so patients should be referred to regional or national services for review and follow-up.

This patient underwent genetic testing and was found to have a mutation in the folliculin gene (FLCN) consistent with Birt–Hogg–Dubé syndrome.

She had genetic counselling and has been enrolled into regular lifelong screening for renal tumours (with annual MRI or ultrasound scanning). Her family members have been offered genetic testing to allow them to be identified early (prior to pneumothorax presentation) and screened for renal tumours.

In the UK, respiratory physicians (as well as geneticists) are permitted to request genetic testing (under code R190, familial pneumothorax) if there is a strong family history or atypical cysts on CT.

e. Should we screen all patients for underlying conditions?

There are data to suggest that patients with presumed sporadic primary pneumothorax (without a strong family history) with a large number or size

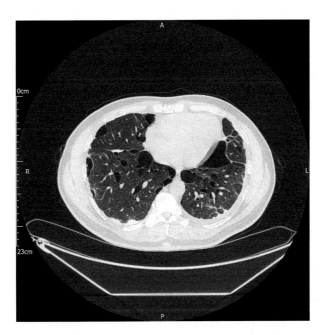

Figure 22.1 Computed tomography (CT) scan for the chest showing irregular paramediastinal and subpleural cysts with lower zone predominance commonly seen in Birt–Hogg–Dubé syndrome (BHD) syndrome.

of blebs (paraseptal cysts) may be at higher risk of recurrence (17). However, other studies have not consistently shown an increased risk or a bleb 'risk score' proven to predict future pneumothorax recurrence (18–22). Therefore, routine CT scanning is not currently justified.

CT scanning should be conducted in those patients with strong family history and considered in any young female patient with PSP, given the relative infrequency of primary pneumothorax in young females and the high female preponderance for LAM (an important diagnosis to make).

## KEY POINTS

- About one in ten patients with spontaneous pneumothorax will have a family history of pneumothorax.
- Patients should be examined for features of familial conditions associated with pneumothorax.
- CT scanning should be conducted in those with a strong family history and considered in any young female patient with spontaneous pneumothorax.
- Genetic testing should be conducted in those patients with a strong family history or features on examination suggestive of an associated condition.
- The long-term risks of further spontaneous pneumothorax or pneumomediastinum are not known.

# REFERENCES

1. Abolnik IZ, Lossos IS, Zlotogora J, Brauer R. On the inheritance of primary spontaneous pneumothorax. *Am J Med Genet* 1991;40(2):155–8.
2. Ren HZ, Zhu CC, Yang C, Chen SL, Xie J, Hou YY, et al. Mutation analysis of the FLCN gene in Chinese patients with sporadic and familial isolated primary spontaneous pneumothorax. *Clin Genet* 2008;74(2):178–83.
3. Hallifax RJ, McKeown E, Sivakumar P, Fairbairn I, Peter C, Leitch A, et al. Ambulatory management of primary spontaneous pneumothorax: An open-label, randomised controlled trial. *Lancet* 2020;396(10243):39–49.
4. Boone PM, Scott RM, Marciniak SJ, Henske EP, Raby BA. The genetics of pneumothorax. *Am J Respir Crit Care Med* 2019;199(11):1344–57.
5. Nickerson ML, Warren MB, Toro JR, Matrosova V, Glenn G, Turner M, et al. Mutations in a novel gene lead to kidney tumors, lung wall defects, and benign tumors of the hair follicle in patients with the Birt-Hogg-Dube syndrome. *Cancer Cell* 2002;2(2):157–64.
6. Ryu JH, Moss J, Beck GJ, Lee JC, Brown KK, Chapman JT, et al. The NHLBI lymphangioleiomyomatosis registry: Characteristics of 230 patients at enrollment. *Am J Respir Crit Care Med* 2006;173(1):105–11.
7. Henske EP, McCormack FX. Lymphangioleiomyomatosis – A wolf in sheep's clothing. *J Clin Invest* 2012;122(11):3807–16.
8. Costello LC, Hartman TE, Ryu JH. High frequency of pulmonary lymphangioleiomyomatosis in women with tuberous sclerosis complex. *Mayo Clin Proc* 2000;75(6):591–4.
9. Henske EP, Jozwiak S, Kingswood JC, Sampson JR, Thiele EA. Tuberous sclerosis complex. *Nat Rev Dis Primers* 2016;2:16035.
10. Pope FM, Martin GR, Lichtenstein JR, Penttinen R, Gerson B, Rowe DW, et al. Patients with Ehlers-Danlos syndrome type IV lack type III collagen. *Proc Natl Acad Sci U S A* 1975;72(4):1314–6.
11. Dietz H. *FBN1*- Related Marfan Syndrome. In: Adam MP, Mirzaa GM, Pagon RA, et al., eds. 1993. *GeneReviews®*. Seattle (WA): University of Washington, Seattle; April 18, 2001.
12. Loeys BL, Dietz HC, Braverman AC, Callewaert BL, De Backer J, Devereux RB, et al. The revised Ghent nosology for the Marfan syndrome. *J Med Genet* 2010;47(7):476–85.
13. MacCarrick G, Black JH 3rd, Bowdin S, El-Hamamsy I, Frischmeyer-Guerrerio PA, Guerrerio AL, et al. Loeys-Dietz syndrome: A primer for diagnosis and management. *Genet Med.* 2014;16(8):576–87.
14. Byers PH. Vascular Ehlers-Danlos Syndrome. 1999 Sep 2 [Updated 2019 Feb 21]. In: Adam MP, Mirzaa GM, Pagon RA, et al., editors. GeneReviews® [Internet]. Seattle (WA): University of Washington, Seattle; 1993–2023.

15. Tobino K, Gunji Y, Kurihara M, Kunogi M, Koike K, Tomiyama N, et al. Characteristics of pulmonary cysts in Birt-Hogg-Dube syndrome: Thin-section CT findings of the chest in 12 patients. *Eur J Radiol* 2011;77(3):403–9.

16. Xu W, Xu Z, Liu Y, Zhan Y, Sui X, Feng R, et al. Characterization of CT scans of patients with Birt-Hogg-Dube syndrome compared with those of Chinese patients with non-BHD diffuse cyst lung diseases. *Orphanet J Rare Dis* 2020;15(1):176.

17. Olesen WH, Katballe N, Sindby JE, Titlestad IL, Andersen PE, Lindahl-Jacobsen R, et al. Surgical treatment versus conventional chest tube drainage in primary spontaneous pneumothorax: A randomized controlled trial. *Eur J Cardio Thorac Surg* 2018;54(1):113–21.

18. Sihoe AD, Yim AP, Lee TW, Wan S, Yuen EHY, Wan IYP, et al. Can CT scanning be used to select patients with unilateral primary spontaneous pneumothorax for bilateral surgery? *Chest* 2000;118(2):380–3.

19. Casali C, Stefani A, Ligabue G, Natali P, Aramini B, Torricelli P, et al. Role of blebs and bullae detected by high-resolution computed tomography and recurrent spontaneous pneumothorax. *Ann Thorac Surg* 2013;95(1):249–55.

20. Martínez-Ramos D, Angel-Yepes V, Escrig-Sos J, Miralles-Tena JM, Salvador-Sanchís JL. Usefulness of computed tomography in determining risk of recurrence after a first episode of primary spontaneous pneumothorax: Therapeutic implications. *Arch Bronconeumol* 2007;43(6):304–8.

21. Huang TW, Lee SC, Cheng YL, Tzao C, Hsu HH, Chang H, et al. Contralateral recurrence of primary spontaneous pneumothorax. *Chest* 2007;132(4):1146–50.

22. Ouanes-Besbes L, Golli M, Knani J, Dachraouia F, Nciria N, El Atrousa S, et al. Prediction of recurrent spontaneous pneumothorax: CT scan findings versus management features. *Respir Med* 2007;101(2):230–6.

# 23

# Post-effusion drainage complication in an 86-year-old woman

POPPY DENNISTON

An 86-year-old patient presented with cough and breathlessness over 3 months but worse over the past few weeks. She had lost 5 kg in weight and had a reduced appetite. She had no lumps or bumps, changes in bladder or bowels, fevers or night sweats. She had a history of previous transient global amnesia and hypertension. There was no previous history of cancer. Medications included losartan, atorvastatin and aspirin. She was normally fit, but now had an ECOG performance status of 3 due to breathlessness. She was an ex-smoker with a 5 pack-year history, and worked as a secretary but was now retired. There was no known history of asbestos exposure, and her husband did not work with asbestos.

On examination, there was no clubbing or cervical lymphadenopathy, but there was minimal pitting oedema and normal heart sounds. Auscultation of the lung fields revealed quiet breath sounds on the right. Breast examination was normal. The initial chest X-ray is shown in Figure 23.1.

a) What is the differential diagnosis and what are the next steps?
   1) Malignancy is the most likely diagnosis, including lung cancer, primary pleural malignancy such as mesothelioma, or metastatic cancer that has spread to the pleura.
   2) Infection should be considered but is unlikely given the lack of fevers or night sweats, and normal inflammatory markers.
   3) Heart failure, or fluid overload, is possible given mild pitting oedema, but given the asymmetrical effusion, we should proceed to pleural sampling.

DOI: 10.1201/9781003081630-23

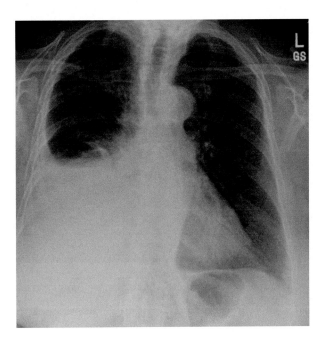

Figure 23.1 Chest X-ray showing a moderate right-sided pleural effusion.

The patient attended for a diagnostic and therapeutic pleural aspiration. Under ultrasound (US) guidance, 1,500 mL of straw-coloured fluid was drained and sent for biochemical, microbiological and cytological analysis. Total protein was 41 g/dL, LDH 482 IU/L and glucose 4.1 mmol/L. MCS was negative. Cytology demonstrated lymphocytes and neutrophils with three-dimensional clusters of mildly atypical epithelioid cells and no loss of nuclear BAP1 staining.

Chest X-ray following pleural aspiration appeared normal. A staging CT chest–abdomen–pelvis to further investigate the cause of the exudative lymphocytic effusion demonstrated a large hydropneumothorax and mediastinal shift (Figure 23.2).

b) What could have caused the CT appearances?
1) *Trauma to the lung during aspiration* – Given the size of the effusion and that the procedure was performed under direct US guidance, this is unlikely. Direct US guidance and performance of aspiration by more experienced proceduralists have been shown to reduce the risk of traumatic pneumothorax during pleural aspiration (1).
2) *Introduction of air during the aspiration* – The introduction of a small amount of air during the pleural procedure is common. It would be unusual to introduce this volume of air, however.
3) *Non-expansile lung (NEL)* – This is the most likely cause for the CT appearances. Here there is a mediastinal shift radiologically, but this is

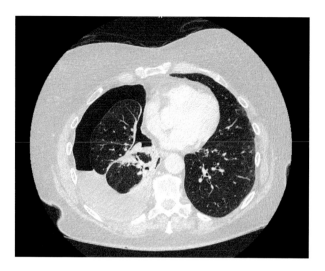

Figure 23.2 Thoracic CT showing right-sided hydropneumothorax and shift of mediastinum to the left.

likely to occur due to physiologically normal negative pleural pressure on the left, with positive pressure on the right due to the presence of air and fluid. The patient ought to be reviewed clinically, but in the absence of a clinical mediastinal shift or physiological disturbance, this is unlikely to need further intervention.

c) How can NEL be defined? What are the main clinical implications of NEL in this case?

NEL has varying definitions in clinical and research practice. Clinically, it is diagnosed by symptoms of cough or chest tightness during drainage, or negative pressure physiology during drainage. Radiological definitions range from the presence of air or fluid in 25%–50% of the hemithorax on chest X-ray (2).

It should be noted that pleural drainage still relieves breathlessness in patients with trapped lung, and so intervention should be a part of palliative measures (3). Pleurodesis will not be possible as pleural apposition is not achievable, and so an indwelling pleural catheter (IPC) would be recommended for long-term fluid management. In select patients, surgical treatment of NEL may be considered.

The patient re-accumulated fluid and given the cytology was non-diagnostic but suspicious, and the CT demonstrated no other site of disease, a local anaesthetic thoracoscopy (LAT) with biopsies and IPC insertion for definitive fluid management was conducted. A diagnosis of epithelioid mesothelioma was confirmed on LAT pleural biopsies.

d) Can we predict NEL?

NEL means talc pleurodesis cannot be attempted, however, it may be concealed until drainage. It would be very helpful to predict NEL in suspected malignant pleural effusion so patients could be offered a 'one-stop shop' of diagnosis and definitive fluid management. This would be particularly useful in patients who are unlikely to be fit enough for systemic anticancer treatment, and therefore in whom histological diagnosis is not essential. Prediction of NEL prior to drainage is therefore a common research question.

Pre-aspiration prediction of NEL based on CT findings may be attempted. The presence of an obstructing bronchial lesion, significant visceral pleural thickening or a very loculated or septated pleural space may predict NEL. Thoracic ultrasound has been proposed as a method of predicting trapped lung. Images obtained during breath-hold may be analysed using M-mode and speckle tracing to detect motion and strain of the cardiac impulse with a sensitivity/specificity of 50%/85% and 71%/85%, respectively (4).

Intra-drainage manometry has been suggested to predict NEL. Elevated pleural elastance correlates with chest radiograph findings of incomplete lung expansion after complete drainage, but the relationship is not absolute. In one study, 34% of patients with normal pleural elastance had incomplete expansion on post-procedure radiographs (5). High pleural elastance may predict NEL with 100% sensitivity and 67% specificity.

Despite these advances in innovative US and pleural manometry, routine practice is to perform a chest radiograph following therapeutic pleural aspiration for suspected malignant pleural effusion (MPE), as it helps to guide further management of MPE. This has poor sensitivity, as reflected in many pleural intervention trials: 13% and 7% of recruited patients were excluded from IPC-PLUS and TAPPS trials despite NEL being a specific exclusion criterion (6,7). This is likely because initial therapeutic thoracentesis is often not complete: some fluid is left behind to allow for future diagnostics such as thoracoscopy or to prevent procedural complications such as re-expansion pulmonary oedema. Therefore, pneumothorax ex vacuo is rare following the initial aspiration.

In practice, therefore, NEL is diagnosed based on symptoms of chest tightness and cough during aspiration, negative pressure physiology with fluid being sucked back into the chest during aspiration, and radiological evidence of pneumothorax ex vacuo.

## KEY POINTS

- Trapped lung is an important entity to recognise and should be differentiated from ongoing air leak and pneumothorax due to visceral pleural damage, either iatrogenic or due to negative pressure, drainage or an underlying disease.

- NEL is variously defined but critically should be used to predict where pleurodesis will not likely be successful, leading to alternative treatment (IPC or repeat pleural aspiration).
- Despite the lack of lung expansion, fluid accumulation in NEL is associated with significant symptoms, and initial drainage to assess symptom relief is indicated.

## REFERENCES

1. Gordon CE, Feller-Kopman D, Balk EM, Smetana GW. Pneumothorax following thoracentesis: A systematic review and meta-analysis. *Arch Intern Med*. 2010;170(4):332–339. doi:10.1001/archinternmed.2009.548
2. Huggins JT, Maldonado F, Chopra A, Rahman N, Light R. Unexpandable lung from pleural disease. *Respirology*. 2018;23(2):160–167. doi:10.1111/resp.13199
3. Muruganandan S, Azzopardi M, Thomas R, et al. The Pleural Effusion And Symptom Evaluation (PLEASE) study of breathlessness in patients with a symptomatic pleural effusion. *Eur Respir J*. 2020;55(5):1900980.
4. Salamonsen MR, Lo AKC, Ng ACT, Bashirzadeh F, Wang WYS, Fielding DIK. Novel use of pleural ultrasound can identify malignant entrapped lung prior to effusion drainage. *Chest*. 2014;146(5):1286–1293.
5. Chopra A, Judson MA, Doelken P, Maldonado F, Rahman NM, Huggins JT. The relationship of pleural manometry with postthoracentesis chest radiographic findings in malignant pleural effusion. *Chest*. 2020;157(2):421–426.
6. Bhatnagar R, Keenan EK, Morley AJ, et al. Outpatient talc administration by indwelling pleural catheter for malignant effusion. *N Engl J Med*. 2018;378(14):1313–1322. doi:10.1056/NEJMoa1716883
7. Bhatnagar R, Piotrowska HEG, Laskawiec-Szkonter M, et al. Effect of thoracoscopic talc poudrage vs talc slurry via chest tube on pleurodesis failure rate among patients with malignant pleural effusions: A randomized clinical trial. *JAMA*. 2020;323(1):60–69. doi:10.1001/jama.2019.19997

# 24

# Chest pain in a 65-year-old writer following pleural fluid aspiration

SOUMYA GHATAK AND RADHIKA BANKA

A 65-year-old male writer presented to the outpatient department with complaints of dry cough and intermittent dull aching chest pain for the past 2 months. He complained of progressive shortness of breath, initially mMRC grade 1 which progressed to mMRC grade 3 over 2 months. He was diagnosed with chronic myeloid leukaemia for which he was being treated with dasatinib 140 mg once daily for the past 1.5 years.

On examination, physiological parameters were stable with significantly reduced breath sounds on auscultation at both lung bases. A chest radiograph revealed moderate-sized bilateral pleural effusions (Figure 24.1).

The patient underwent an ultrasound-guided diagnostic and therapeutic pleural aspiration of the right-sided effusion during which 1.8 litres of serosanguinous fluid was aspirated.

Immediately after the drainage procedure, he complained of acute central chest pain, breathlessness and cough with pink frothy sputum. Vital signs at this point were HR 110/min, BP 110/70, RR 30/min and oxygen saturations of 85% on room air.

He was therefore admitted to the intensive care unit (ICU) and an immediate chest X-ray was conducted (Figure 24.2).

a. What does the chest X-ray show? What is the diagnosis?

   The chest X-ray shows right-sided lower zone haziness with a moderate left pleural effusion. Given the clinical picture, the diagnosis is consistent with re-expansion pulmonary oedema after pleural fluid aspiration.

DOI: 10.1201/9781003081630-24                                                                147

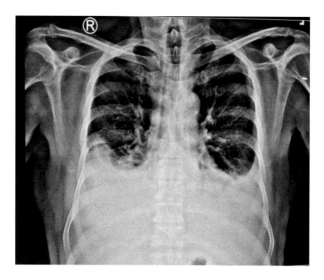

Figure 24.1 Chest radiograph showing moderate-sized bilateral pleural effusions.

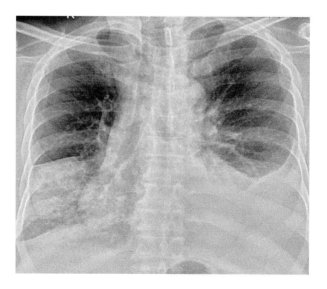

Figure 24.2 Chest radiograph showing right-sided lower zone haziness with a moderate left pleural effusion.

b. What is re-expansion pulmonary oedema?

Re-expansion pulmonary oedema (REPO) is a rare type of non-cardiogenic pulmonary oedema which is most commonly observed as an iatrogenic adverse event following the evacuation of a significant amount of pleural effusion or pneumothorax. It is typically unilateral but can be bilateral following a unilateral intervention. In the majority of studies, the reported incidence after pneumothorax and pleural effusion drainage range between 0% and 1% (1). Although rare, this condition has a mortality rate of nearly 20% (2).

c. What is the pathophysiology behind REPO?

The mechanism of REPO is highly heterogeneous and poorly understood. One of the more intriguing hypotheses suggests that inflammation-induced increased pulmonary capillary permeability is the primary cause (2).

An inflammatory reaction secondary to the generation of reactive oxygen species and superoxide radicals is hypothesised to be the key reason for REPO; this occurs due to sudden ventilation and perfusion in chronically hypoxic alveolar cells in atelectatic lung during fluid or air evacuation. This cascade of events eventually causes a rise in capillary permeability. Inflammatory mediators such as interleukin 8, leukotriene B4 and monocyte chemotactic activating factor have been found in both animal and human cases of REPO (3).

As an alternative hypothesis, certain studies point to alternate mechanisms that may cause REPO in certain groups. These include increased pulmonary hydrostatic pressure due to enhanced venous return as well as pressure-induced mechanical damage of the alveolar capillaries associated with reduced levels of functional surfactant resulting in increased pressure through the capillary–alveolar membrane coupled with altered lymphatic clearance (4).

d. What is the presentation of the condition?

Chest discomfort, a persistent severe cough most commonly associated with foamy sputum and dyspnoea after aspiration are all cardinal symptoms of REPO. In 64% of patients, symptoms begin within 1–2 hours of lung re-expansion, and in almost all of them symptoms occur within the first 24 hours after aspiration (4). On examination, the patient is typically tachycardic, tachypnoeic with hypoxemia which may be refractory to oxygen therapy. On auscultation, crackles are found in the affected hemithorax. Chest radiograph and CT thorax findings mimic pulmonary oedema and show the presence of unilateral haziness, which can occasionally be bilateral or rarely affect only the contralateral lung (5).

e. What are the risk factors to develop REPO?

REPO is more commonly seen following pneumothorax drainage as compared to pleural fluid aspiration. The risk of developing REPO increases with an increased duration and size of the pneumothorax. Between 20 and 40 years old, prolonged lung collapse (more than 72 hours), the use of elevated negative pressures during thoracic drainage (more than 20 cm $H_2O$), and rapid lung expansion with a substantial volume of pleural fluid drainage (more than 1.5 L) are risk factors established via various studies (6, 7, 8).

The pleural fluid from the aspiration was demonstrated to be a borderline exudative (protein 3 g/dl, glucose 5.6 mmol/L, LDH 96 U/L) with negative adenosine deaminase (ADA) and no evidence of infective aetiology. The fluid cytology was negative and the flow cytometry did not reveal any atypical cells.

The patient was started on a high-flow nasal cannula in the ICU and one dose of intravenous diuretic was given. Over the next 24 hours, he recovered completely with no supplemental oxygen requirement. Since he complained of persistent dyspnoea, contralateral thoracentesis was performed under close monitoring and 1 litre of pleural fluid was drained over 36 hours (Figure 24.3). Since he remained hemodynamically stable, he was discharged the following day.

f. What is the treatment for REPO?

For REPO to be effectively managed, prompt identification is critical. Supportive treatment is the standard of care but depends on the severity of presentation (8). Patients with mild symptoms might benefit from oxygen supplementation alone, but those with significant symptoms may necessitate endotracheal intubation and mechanical ventilation. Bi-level positive airway pressure and non-invasive ventilation may assist patients with worsening symptoms and avoid the need for endotracheal intubation (9). Diuretics, bronchodilators, prostaglandin analogues (like misoprostol), ibuprofen and

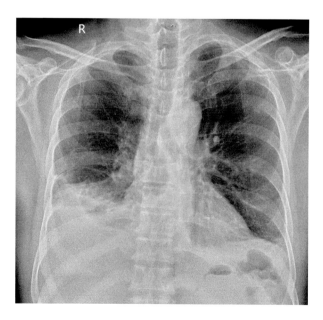

Figure 24.3 Chest radiograph showing partial resolution of right pleural effusion with complete resolution of left pleural effusion.

steroids have been used, although most of the evidence regarding them is anecdotal in origin (10).

g. What are the measures needed to prevent REPO?

Although the risks of developing REPO remain highly uncertain given its rarity, the British Thoracic Society's 2023 pleural guidelines state a limit of 1.5 litres of fluid aspiration in one attempt to prevent the condition in general. It is recognised that larger volumes than this can be aspirated with close monitoring. The guidelines direct an immediate stoppage of aspiration if the patient develops a cough, dyspnoea or a drop in saturation (11). Some authorities recommend constant measurement of intrapleural pressures by pleural manometry during thoracentesis and stopping the procedure when the intrapleural pressure falls below –20 cm of Hg (1, 10, 12, 13), although there is no evidence that this prevents REPO.

## KEY POINTS

- REPO can be seen after a pleural aspiration or pneumothorax drainage. Although rare, can be associated with high mortality.
- Diagnosis of REPO should be suspected when large-volume thoracocentesis is performed with the patient complaining of dyspnoea, cough or chest pain following the procedure.
- The authors recommend a maximum of 1.5 litres of pleural fluid drainage in one setting unless the patient is closely monitored.
- Management is similar to that of pulmonary oedema: supplemental oxygen, and diuretics with or without positive pressure ventilation.

## REFERENCES

1. Feller-Kopman D, Berkowitz D, Boiselle P, Ernst A. Large-volume thoracentesis and the risk of reexpansion pulmonary edema. *Ann Thorac Surg* 2007;84(5):1656–61.
2. Sherman SC. Reexpansion pulmonary edema: A case report and review of the current literature. *J Emerg Med* 2003;24(1):23–7.
3. Jackson RM, Veal CF, Alexander CB, et al. Re-expansion pulmonary edema. A potential role for free radicals in its pathogenesis. *Am Rev Respir Dis* 1988;137(5):1165–71.
4. Mahfood S, Hix WR, Aaron BL, et al. Reexpansion pulmonary edema. *Ann Thorac Surg* 1988;45(3):340–5.
5. Ragozzino MW, Greene R. Bilateral reexpansion pulmonary edema following unilateral pleurocentesis. *Chest* 1991;99(2):506–8.
6. Matsuura Y, Nomimura T, Murakami H, et al. Clinical analysis of reexpansion pulmonary edema. *Chest* 1991;100(6):1562–6.
7. Taira N, Kawabata T, Ichi T, Yohena T, Kawasaki H, Ishikawa K. An analysis of and new risk factors for reexpansion pulmonary edema following spontaneous pneumothorax. *J Thorac Dis* 2014 September;6(9):1187–92.

8. Morioka H, Takada K, Matsumoto S, Kojima E, Iwata S, Okachi S. Re-expansion pulmonary edema: Evaluation of risk factors in 173 episodes of spontaneous pneumothorax. *Respir Investig* 2013;51(1):35–9.

9. Sawafuji M, Ishizaka A, Kohno M, et al. Role of Rho-kinase in reexpansion pulmonary edema in rabbits. *Am J Physiol Lung Cell Mol Physiol* 2005;289(6):L946–L53.

10. Iqbal M, Multz AS, Rossoff LJ, et al. Reexpansion pulmonary edema after VATS successfully treated with continuous positive airway pressure. *Ann Thorac Surg* 2000;70(2):669–71.

11. Roberts ME, Rahman NM, Maskell NA, et al. British Thoracic Society Guideline for pleural disease. *Thorax.* 2023);78(Suppl 3):s1–s42.

12. Feller-Kopman D, Parker MJ, Schwartzstein RM. Assessment of pleural pressure in the evaluation of pleural effusions. *Chest* 2009;135(1):201–9.

13. Havelock T, Teoh R, Laws D, et al. Pleural procedures and thoracic ultrasound: British Thoracic Society Pleural Disease Guideline 2010. *Thorax* 2010;65 (Suppl 2):ii61–ii76.

14. British Thoracic Society. British Thoracic Society. (2022). BTS guideline for pleural disease [pleuralguidelines2022]. https://www.brit-thoracic.org.uk/qualityimprovement/guidelines/pleural-disease/.

# 25

# A simple pneumothorax?

RACHEL MERCER

A 20-year-old man presented to the emergency department with chest pain. The pain originally occurred when playing sport a few days prior, then worsened with repeat activity precipitating an admission to the emergency department. The pain was pleuritic in nature and there was associated shortness of breath. There was no significant past medical history; he was a social smoker and lived with several housemates.

Observations on admission showed a heart rate of 108 beats per minute, saturations of 98% on air with a respiratory rate of 20 and blood pressure of 148/78 mmHg. He was apyrexial. A chest radiograph demonstrated a right-sided pneumothorax which was 2 cm in depth at the hilum along with a small right pleural effusion.

a) What are the management options for this patient?

There are several options for this gentleman as he does not display any high-risk characteristics (no haemodynamic compromise, significant hypoxia, bilateral pneumothoraces, underlying lung disease and the patient is young without a significant smoking history) (1).

It would thus be reasonable to consider either conservative management or intervention. If the patient opted for intervention, needle aspiration or ambulatory treatment (using an integrated drainage device and Heimlich valve, such as a pleural vent device) are the initial management options.

The chest X-ray is shown in Figure 25.1. The patient expressed a preference for intervention.

b) Would you have any concerns about undertaking a needle aspiration or inserting a pleural vent for this patient?

Although the lung can be seen just behind the area of the second intercostal space, this is not a contraindication to undertaking an aspiration or

DOI: 10.1201/9781003081630-25

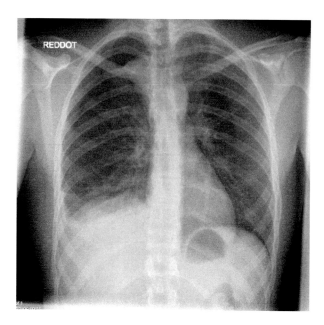

Figure 25.1 Chest X-ray showing a small right-sided hydropneumothorax.

pleural vent insertion, as this is a two-dimensional image and there is likely to be sufficient space for insertion of the needle. An aspiration can also be undertaken in the axilla (safe triangle) where there is a clear space for intervention.

Small pleural effusions are common in patients presenting with a pneumothorax and can be reactive or evidence of a small amount of bleeding.

A needle aspiration was undertaken and 2.5 L of air was aspirated. A repeat chest X-ray was undertaken which showed an increase in the size of the pneumothorax (Figure 25.2). In view of this, a chest drain was inserted (Figure 25.3). The patient's heart rate had increased to 120/min and blood pressure had reduced to 100/50 mmHg. At this point, a CT scan was organised (Figure 25.4).

c) What does the radiology show?

The effusion seems to have increased markedly in size; with the new tachycardia, there is a concern about pleural bleeding leading to hypovolaemia. The tip of the chest drain is very deep and it is not clear whether this represents an iatrogenic injury or the drain is within the fissure. This may mean that the drain is not functioning to relieve the pneumothorax.

The patient was examined and noted to be pale and clammy. The chest drain bottle contained 2 L of blood of heavily blood-stained fluid.

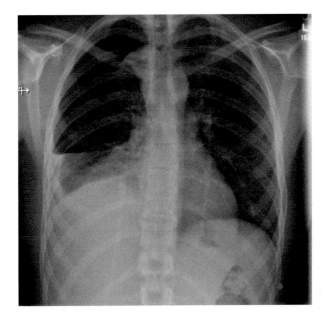

Figure 25.2 Chest X-ray showing an increase in the size of right-sided hydropneumothorax.

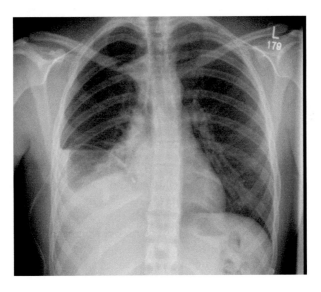

Figure 25.3 Chest X-ray showing the presence of a right-sided hydropneumo-thorax with drain in situ.

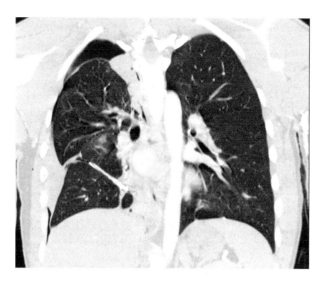

Figure 25.4 Coronal view of CT thorax showing the presence of a small, right-sided pneumothorax with deep insertion of an intercostal chest drain (ICD).

d) How would you proceed in managing this patient and how would you manage the chest drain?

The patient appears to be in shock and should be managed using the ABCDE approach. The patient should be given oxygen, and two wide-bore cannulas should be inserted. A sample from the pleural fluid should be undertaken to confirm the diagnosis of a haemothorax (haematocrit of >50% of the serum). The patient should be fluid resuscitated including with blood transfusions. The patient is likely to need intervention in the form of radiology or thoracic surgery and the relevant services should be urgently contacted along with contacting the critical care team (2, 3).

Removing the chest drain should not be undertaken at this point, as it will not stop the bleeding. There are a number of factors which could be considered when determining whether the chest drain should be clamped. If the patient has a pleural bleed, then clamping the drain is unlikely to tamponade the bleeding as the chest cavity is a large volume area. Apposition of the lung to the chest wall may aid in stopping the bleeding, but this would not occur if the drain was clamped. The patient may also have an ongoing air leak which could compromise them further if the drain was clamped. If the bleeding was due to the chest drain incorrectly inserted into the lung and accessing a vessel, then clamping the drain may be the correct action.

e) What do you think was the cause of the bleeding?

The patient had a reasonably sized effusion prior to any intervention; this makes it more likely that the bleeding occurred when the pneumothorax developed (via tearing of an adhesion) rather than an iatrogenic cause. The patient was transferred for thoracic surgery and on direct examination of the thoracic cavity there was no evidence that the drain had caused any damage and a remnant of an adhesion at the apex was noted.

## KEY POINTS

- Pneumothorax is often associated with a small amount of intrapleural bleeding which is normally self-limiting and due to tearing of adhesions as the lung collapses away from the chest wall.
- In any patient post-pleural intervention with tachycardia or hypotension, pleural haemorrhage should be considered.
- Urgent resuscitation should be instituted, and immediate radiology (preferably ultrasound at the bedside and contrast CT) should be conducted.
- Treatment options include thoracic surgery and interventional radiology, which should be contacted as soon as the diagnosis is confirmed.

## REFERENCES

1. Roberts ME, Rahman NM, Maskell NA, et al. British Thoracic Society Guideline for pleural disease. *Thorax.* 2023;78(Suppl 3):s1–s42.
2. Ng CSH, Wong RHL, Wan IYP, et al. Spontaneous Haemopneumothorax: Current Management. *Postgraduate Medical Journal.* 2011;87(1031):630–635.
3. Sundaralingam A, Bedawi EO, Harriss EK, Munavvar M, Rahman NM. The Frequency, Risk Factors, and Management of Complications From Pleural Procedures. *Chest.* 2022;161(5):1407–1425.

# Index

## A

ABP, *see* Autologous blood patch
    pleurodesis
Abram's needle, 44
Adenosine deaminase (ADA), 42
Ambulatory Heimlich valve, 119, 120
Amiodarone-related effusion, 85, 86
Anti-tubercular treatment, 44
Autologous blood patch pleurodesis
    (ABP), 120

## B

Benign asbestos pleural effusion (BAPE),
    27, 67, 68
Bilateral transudative effusions, 46–50
Biliothorax, 93
Birt–Hogg–Dube (BHD) syndrome,
    137–139

## C

Chemical pleurodesis, 119–120
Chronic pleural inflammation, 27
Chylothorax, 103
    causes, 72
    diagnosis, 72–73
    management, 73–74
Clagett thoracotomy, 31

## D

Dasatinib-induced pleural effusion, 110
Drug-induced pleuritis, 87
Drug-resistant TPE, 44

## E

Eosinophilic pleural effusion, 87, 129
Epithelioid mesothelioma, 18, 144

## G

Gorham–Stout disease (GSD), 103–105

## H

Hepatic hydrothorax (HH), 58–60
    non-pleural options, management
        of, 60
    pleural options, treatment of, 60–62

## I

IgG4-related disease (IgG4-RD)
    diagnosis, 95–97
    pericarditis, 96
    treatment, 98
Indwelling pleural catheters (IPCs), 13–16,
    19, 26, 27, 30, 50, 55, 60, 61, 144

IPC-related pleural space infection, 28–29
in malignant pleural effusion, 49
role in septated MPE, 19–20
Intra-drainage manometry, 145
Intrapleural fibrinolytic therapy, 21–22
IPC, *see* Indwelling pleural catheter placement

## L

LAT, *see* Local anaesthetic thoracoscopy
Light's criteria, 2–3
Local anaesthetic thoracoscopy (LAT), 4, 131, 144
Loeys–Dietz syndrome, 137
Lymphangioleiomyomatosis (LAM), 39, 137, 138

## M

Macklin effect, 125
Malignant pleural effusion (MPE), 10, 145
diagnosis, 11, 13
imaging, 11
pleurodesis, 13–15
Medical thoracoscopy, 13, 38
evaluating undifferentiated pleural effusions, 67
Mesothelioma, 15–16
MIST-1 RCT, 38
MPE, *see* Malignant pleural effusion
Mycobacterium tuberculosis (MTB), 42, 43

## N

NEL, *see* Non-expansile lung
Non-expansile lung (NEL), 143–144
clinical implications, 144
prediction, 145
Non-specific pleuritis (NSP), 4–5
causes, 5
malignant process, 5–6
NSP, *see* Non-specific pleuritis

## P

PAL, *see* Persistent air leak
PD-associated pleuroperitoneal leak
management, 55
monitoring patient with, 54
Persistent air leak (PAL), 118–120
PET/CT, 113
malignant pleural effusion, 11
Pleural biopsy, 32, 44, 80–81, 87, 97
Pleural Effusion and Symptom Evaluation (PLEASE) study, 107
Pleural infection, 34, 38
clinical predictors of development, 35
Pleural thickening
diagnosis, 80
Pleurodesis, 13–15
Pneumomediastinum, 124–126
Post-effusion drainage complication, 142–145
Primary spontaneous pneumothorax (PSP), 116, 136

## R

RAPID score, 35, 36
Recurrent pneumothoraces, 136–139
REDUCE study, 49
Re-expansion pulmonary oedema (REPO), 148–149
pathophysiology, 149
presentation, 149
preventive measures, 151
risk factors, 149
treatment, 150–151
REPO, *see* Re-expansion pulmonary oedema
Rheumatoid pleuritis, 27

## S

Secondary spontaneous pneumothorax (SSP), 116, 119
Septated malignant pleural effusion

diagnosis, 18–19
intrapleural fibrinolytic therapy, 21–22
pleural infection, 20
role of IPCs in, 19–20
SFTP, *see* Solitary fibrous tumour of the
pleura
Solitary fibrous tumour of the pleura
(SFTP), 10, 112–114
management, 114
Solitary pleural nodule, 113–114
SSP, *see* Secondary spontaneous
pneumothorax

## T

Talc pleurodesis, 49
TE, *see* Thoracic endometriosis
Thoracic endometriosis (TE), 131–133
diagnosis and management, 133–134
Thoracoscopic view, pleural surface, 103, 104
TIME 3 trial, 21

TPE, *see* Tuberculous pleural effusion
Transudative effusion, 48
talc pleurodesis role in, 49
Tuberculous pleural effusion (TPE), 41, 42
treatment, 44
ultrasound-guided and thoracoscopic
biopsies, 44

## U

Ultrasound (US) image
echogenic pleural effusion, 64, 65
septated pleural effusion, 19, 20, 43
Ultrasound-guided pleural biopsy, 18, 44,
114

## V

VATS, *see* Video-assisted thoracoscopic
surgery
Video-assisted thoracoscopic surgery
(VATS), 18, 31, 56, 80, 118, 134

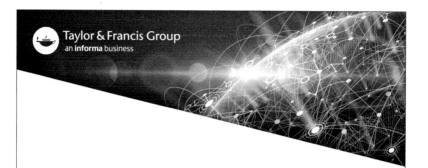